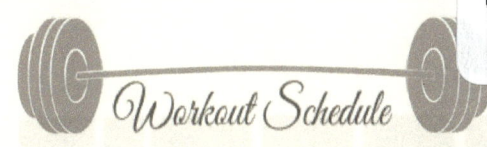

Workout Schedule

NAME: _ _ _ _ _ _ _ DATA: / /

☐ DAY 1

☐ DAY 2

☐ DAY 3

☐ DAY 4

☐ DAY 5

☐ DAY 6

☐ DAY 7

NOTES

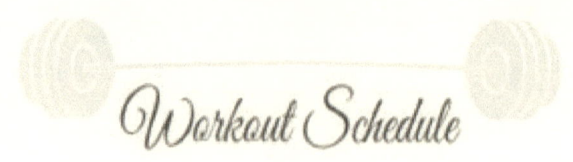

Workout Schedule

Name: _____   Date: _____

Goals: _____

Warm Up

Activity	Sets	Reps	Time	Dist	Intensity	Note

Core Body

Exercises	Sets	Reps	Weight	Rest Time	Note

Upper Body

Exercises	Sets	Reps	Weight	1RM	Rest Time	Note

Lower Body

Exercises	Sets	Reps	Weight	1RM	Rest Time	Note

Cool Down

Activity	Sets	Reps	Time	Dist.	Intensity	Note

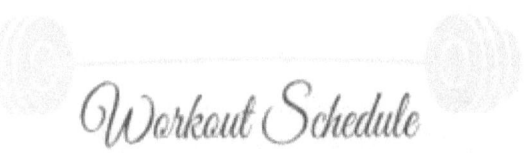

Workout Schedule

Name: Date:

Goals:

Warm Up

Activity	Sets	Reps	Time	Dist	Intensity	Note

Core Body

Exercises	Sets	Reps	Weight	Rest Time	Note

Upper Body

Exercises	Sets	Reps	Weight	1RM	Rest Time	Note

Lower Body

Exercises	Sets	Reps	Weight	1RM	Rest Time	Note

Cool Down

Activity	Sets	Reps	Time	Dist.	Intensity	Note

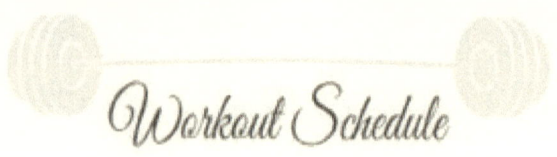

Workout Schedule

Name: _____   Date: _____

Goals: _____

Warm Up

Activity	Sets	Reps	Time	Dist	Intensity	Note

Core Body

Exercises	Sets	Reps	Weight	Rest Time	Note

Upper Body

Exercises	Sets	Reps	Weight	1RM	Rest Time	Note

Lower Body

Exercises	Sets	Reps	Weight	1RM	Rest Time	Note

Cool Down

Activity	Sets	Reps	Time	Dist.	Intensity	Note

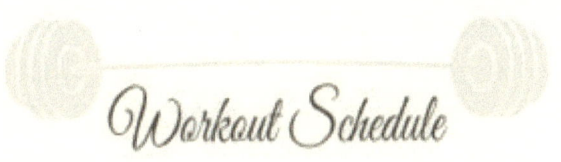

Workout Schedule

Name: _____   Date: _____

Goals: _____

Warm Up

Activity	Sets	Reps	Time	Dist	Intensity	Note

Core Body

Exercises	Sets	Reps	Weight	Rest Time	Note

Upper Body

Exercises	Sets	Reps	Weight	1RM	Rest Time	Note

Lower Body

Exercises	Sets	Reps	Weight	1RM	Rest Time	Note

Cool Down

Activity	Sets	Reps	Time	Dist.	Intensity	Note

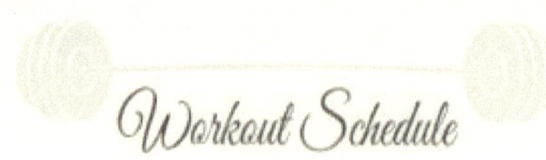

Workout Schedule

Name: _____ Date: _____

Goals: _____

Warm Up

Activity	Sets	Reps	Time	Dist	Intensity	Note

Core Body

Exercises	Sets	Reps	Weight	Rest Time	Note

Upper Body

Exercises	Sets	Reps	Weight	1RM	Rest Time	Note

Lower Body

Exercises	Sets	Reps	Weight	1RM	Rest Time	Note

Cool Down

Activity	Sets	Reps	Time	Dist.	Intensity	Note

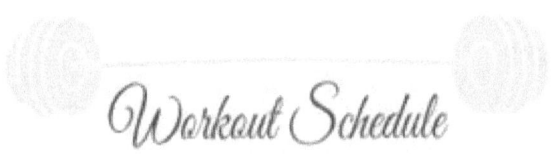

Workout Schedule

Name: Date:

Goals:

Warm Up

Activity	Sets	Reps	Time	Dist	Intensity	Note

Core Body

Exercises	Sets	Reps	Weight	Rest Time	Note

Upper Body

Exercises	Sets	Reps	Weight	1RM	Rest Time	Note

Lower Body

Exercises	Sets	Reps	Weight	1RM	Rest Time	Note

Cool Down

Activity	Sets	Reps	Time	Dist.	Intensity	Note

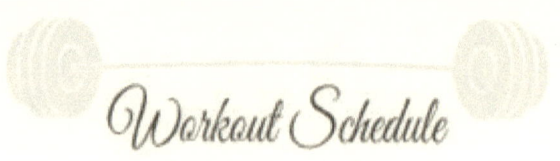

Workout Schedule

Name: _____   Date: _____

Goals: _____

Warm Up

Activity	Sets	Reps	Time	Dist	Intensity	Note

Core Body

Exercises	Sets	Reps	Weight	Rest Time	Note

Upper Body

Exercises	Sets	Reps	Weight	1RM	Rest Time	Note

Lower Body

Exercises	Sets	Reps	Weight	1RM	Rest Time	Note

Cool Down

Activity	Sets	Reps	Time	Dist.	Intensity	Note

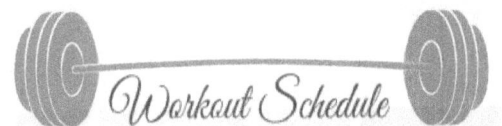

Workout Schedule

NAME: _ _ _ _ _ _ _ _

DATA: / /

☐ DAY 1

☐ DAY 2

☐ DAY 3

☐ DAY 4

☐ DAY 5

☐ DAY 6

☐ DAY 7

NOTES

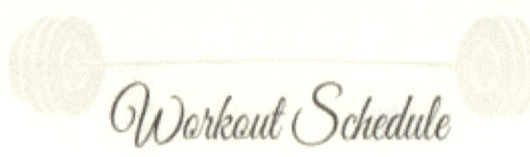

Workout Schedule

Name: Date:

Goals:

Warm Up

Activity	Sets	Reps	Time	Dist	Intensity	Note

Core Body

Exercises	Sets	Reps	Weight	Rest Time	Note

Upper Body

Exercises	Sets	Reps	Weight	1RM	Rest Time	Note

Lower Body

Exercises	Sets	Reps	Weight	1RM	Rest Time	Note

Cool Down

Activity	Sets	Reps	Time	Dist.	Intensity	Note

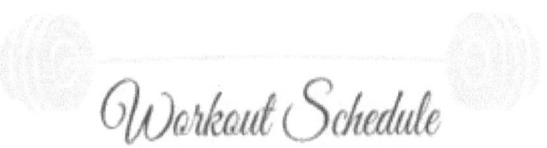

Workout Schedule

Name: Date:

Goals:

Warm Up

Activity	Sets	Reps	Time	Dist	Intensity	Note

Core Body

Exercises	Sets	Reps	Weight	Rest Time	Note

Upper Body

Exercises	Sets	Reps	Weight	1RM	Rest Time	Note

Lower Body

Exercises	Sets	Reps	Weight	1RM	Rest Time	Note

Cool Down

Activity	Sets	Reps	Time	Dist.	Intensity	Note

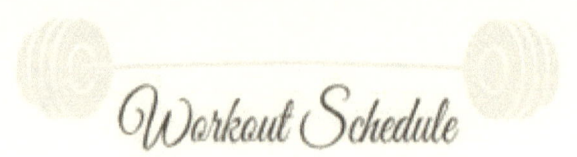

Workout Schedule

Name: _____   **Date:** _____

Goals: _____

Warm Up

Activity	Sets	Reps	Time	Dist	Intensity	Note

Core Body

Exercises	Sets	Reps	Weight	Rest Time	Note

Upper Body

Exercises	Sets	Reps	Weight	1RM	Rest Time	Note

Lower Body

Exercises	Sets	Reps	Weight	1RM	Rest Time	Note

Cool Down

Activity	Sets	Reps	Time	Dist.	Intensity	Note

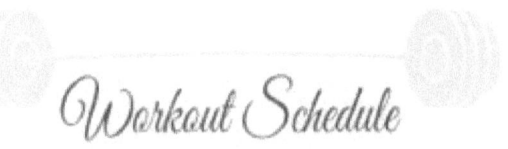

Workout Schedule

Name: Date:

Goals:

Warm Up

Activity	Sets	Reps	Time	Dist	Intensity	Note

Core Body

Exercises	Sets	Reps	Weight	Rest Time	Note

Upper Body

Exercises	Sets	Reps	Weight	1RM	Rest Time	Note

Lower Body

Exercises	Sets	Reps	Weight	1RM	Rest Time	Note

Cool Down

Activity	Sets	Reps	Time	Dist.	Intensity	Note

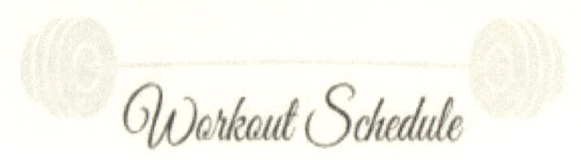

Workout Schedule

Name: _____   Date: _____

Goals: _____

Warm Up

Activity	Sets	Reps	Time	Dist	Intensity	Note

Core Body

Exercises	Sets	Reps	Weight	Rest Time	Note

Upper Body

Exercises	Sets	Reps	Weight	1RM	Rest Time	Note

Lower Body

Exercises	Sets	Reps	Weight	1RM	Rest Time	Note

Cool Down

Activity	Sets	Reps	Time	Dist.	Intensity	Note

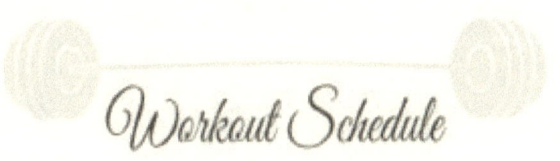

Workout Schedule

Name: _____ Date: _____

Goals: _____

Warm Up

Activity	Sets	Reps	Time	Dist	Intensity	Note

Core Body

Exercises	Sets	Reps	Weight	Rest Time	Note

Upper Body

Exercises	Sets	Reps	Weight	1RM	Rest Time	Note

Lower Body

Exercises	Sets	Reps	Weight	1RM	Rest Time	Note

Cool Down

Activity	Sets	Reps	Time	Dist.	Intensity	Note

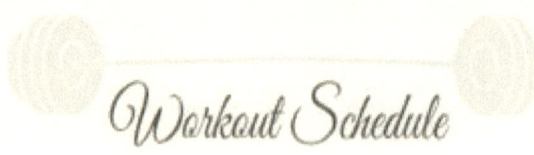

Workout Schedule

Name: _____   Date: _____

Goals: _____

Warm Up

Activity	Sets	Reps	Time	Dist	Intensity	Note

Core Body

Exercises	Sets	Reps	Weight	Rest Time	Note

Upper Body

Exercises	Sets	Reps	Weight	1RM	Rest Time	Note

Lower Body

Exercises	Sets	Reps	Weight	1RM	Rest Time	Note

Cool Down

Activity	Sets	Reps	Time	Dist.	Intensity	Note

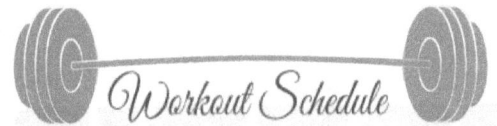

Workout Schedule

NAME: _ _ _ _ _ _ _ _ DATA: / /

☐ DAY 1

☐ DAY 2

☐ DAY 3

☐ DAY 4

☐ DAY 5

☐ DAY 6

☐ DAY 7

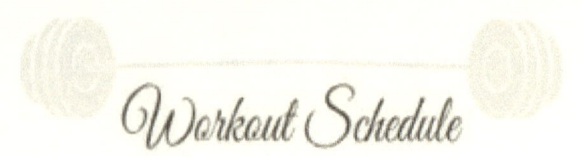

Workout Schedule

Name: _____ Date: _____

Goals: _____

Warm Up

Activity	Sets	Reps	Time	Dist	Intensity	Note

Core Body

Exercises	Sets	Reps	Weight	Rest Time	Note

Upper Body

Exercises	Sets	Reps	Weight	1RM	Rest Time	Note

Lower Body

Exercises	Sets	Reps	Weight	1RM	Rest Time	Note

Cool Down

Activity	Sets	Reps	Time	Dist.	Intensity	Note

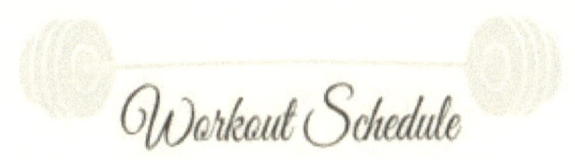

Workout Schedule

Name: _____   Date: _____

Goals: _____

Warm Up

Activity	Sets	Reps	Time	Dist	Intensity	Note

Core Body

Exercises	Sets	Reps	Weight	Rest Time	Note

Upper Body

Exercises	Sets	Reps	Weight	1RM	Rest Time	Note

Lower Body

Exercises	Sets	Reps	Weight	1RM	Rest Time	Note

Cool Down

Activity	Sets	Reps	Time	Dist.	Intensity	Note

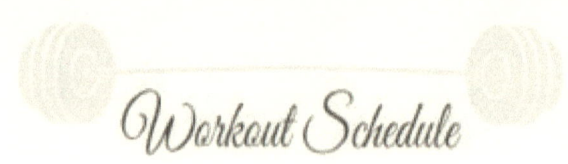

Workout Schedule

Name: _____   Date: _____

Goals: _____

Warm Up

Activity	Sets	Reps	Time	Dist	Intensity	Note

Core Body

Exercises	Sets	Reps	Weight	Rest Time	Note

Upper Body

Exercises	Sets	Reps	Weight	1RM	Rest Time	Note

Lower Body

Exercises	Sets	Reps	Weight	1RM	Rest Time	Note

Cool Down

Activity	Sets	Reps	Time	Dist.	Intensity	Note

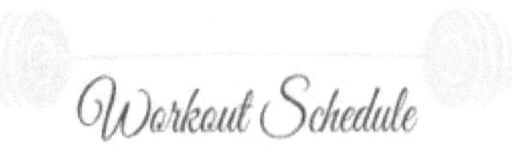

Workout Schedule

Name: Date:

Goals:

Warm Up

Activity	Sets	Reps	Time	Dist	Intensity	Note

Core Body

Exercises	Sets	Reps	Weight	Rest Time	Note

Upper Body

Exercises	Sets	Reps	Weight	1RM	Rest Time	Note

Lower Body

Exercises	Sets	Reps	Weight	1RM	Rest Time	Note

Cool Down

Activity	Sets	Reps	Time	Dist.	Intensity	Note

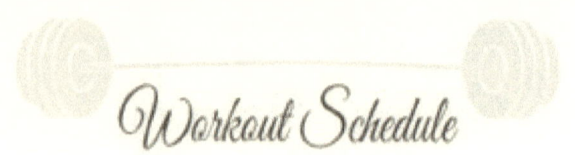

Workout Schedule

Name: _____   Date: _____

Goals: _____

Warm Up

Activity	Sets	Reps	Time	Dist	Intensity	Note

Core Body

Exercises	Sets	Reps	Weight	Rest Time	Note

Upper Body

Exercises	Sets	Reps	Weight	1RM	Rest Time	Note

Lower Body

Exercises	Sets	Reps	Weight	1RM	Rest Time	Note

Cool Down

Activity	Sets	Reps	Time	Dist.	Intensity	Note

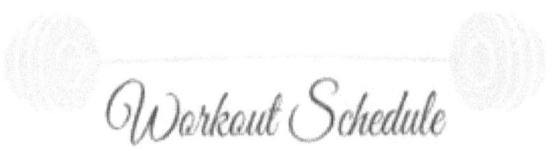

Workout Schedule

Name: Date:

Goals:

Warm Up

Activity	Sets	Reps	Time	Dist	Intensity	Note

Core Body

Exercises	Sets	Reps	Weight	Rest Time	Note

Upper Body

Exercises	Sets	Reps	Weight	1RM	Rest Time	Note

Lower Body

Exercises	Sets	Reps	Weight	1RM	Rest Time	Note

Cool Down

Activity	Sets	Reps	Time	Dist.	Intensity	Note

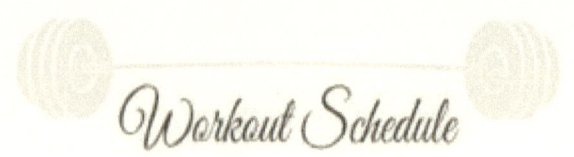

Workout Schedule

Name: _____ Date: _____

Goals: _____

Warm Up

Activity	Sets	Reps	Time	Dist	Intensity	Note

Core Body

Exercises	Sets	Reps	Weight	Rest Time	Note

Upper Body

Exercises	Sets	Reps	Weight	1RM	Rest Time	Note

Lower Body

Exercises	Sets	Reps	Weight	1RM	Rest Time	Note

Cool Down

Activity	Sets	Reps	Time	Dist.	Intensity	Note

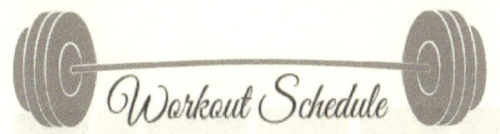

Workout Schedule

NAME: _ _ _ _ _ _ _   DATA: / /

☐ DAY 1

☐ DAY 2

☐ DAY 3

☐ DAY 4

☐ DAY 5

☐ DAY 6

☐ DAY 7

NOTES

○

○

○

○

○

○

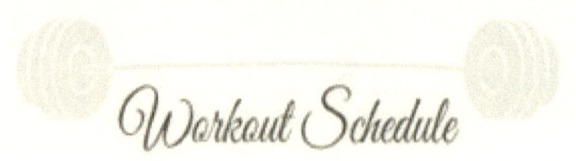

Workout Schedule

Name: _____   **Date:** _____

Goals: _____

Warm Up

Activity	Sets	Reps	Time	Dist	Intensity	Note

Core Body

Exercises	Sets	Reps	Weight	Rest Time	Note

Upper Body

Exercises	Sets	Reps	Weight	1RM	Rest Time	Note

Lower Body

Exercises	Sets	Reps	Weight	1RM	Rest Time	Note

Cool Down

Activity	Sets	Reps	Time	Dist.	Intensity	Note

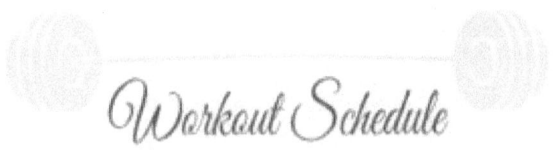

Workout Schedule

Name: Date:

Goals:

Warm Up

Activity	Sets	Reps	Time	Dist	Intensity	Note

Core Body

Exercises	Sets	Reps	Weight	Rest Time	Note

Upper Body

Exercises	Sets	Reps	Weight	1RM	Rest Time	Note

Lower Body

Exercises	Sets	Reps	Weight	1RM	Rest Time	Note

Cool Down

Activity	Sets	Reps	Time	Dist.	Intensity	Note

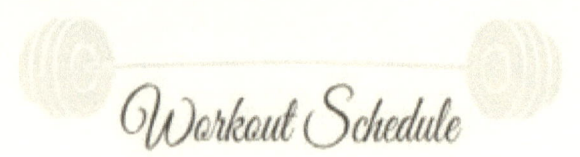

Workout Schedule

Name: _____   Date: _____

Goals: _____

Warm Up

Activity	Sets	Reps	Time	Dist	Intensity	Note

Core Body

Exercises	Sets	Reps	Weight	Rest Time	Note

Upper Body

Exercises	Sets	Reps	Weight	1RM	Rest Time	Note

Lower Body

Exercises	Sets	Reps	Weight	1RM	Rest Time	Note

Cool Down

Activity	Sets	Reps	Time	Dist.	Intensity	Note

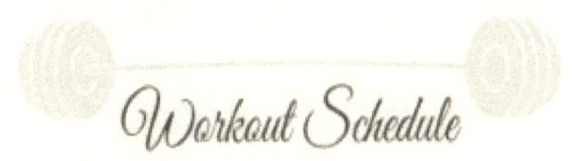

Workout Schedule

Name: _____   Date: _____

Goals: _____

Warm Up

Activity	Sets	Reps	Time	Dist	Intensity	Note

Core Body

Exercises	Sets	Reps	Weight	Rest Time	Note

Upper Body

Exercises	Sets	Reps	Weight	1RM	Rest Time	Note

Lower Body

Exercises	Sets	Reps	Weight	1RM	Rest Time	Note

Cool Down

Activity	Sets	Reps	Time	Dist.	Intensity	Note

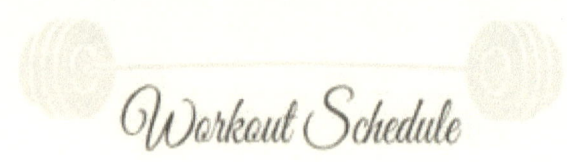

Workout Schedule

Name: _____   Date: _____

Goals: _____

Warm Up

Activity	Sets	Reps	Time	Dist	Intensity	Note

Core Body

Exercises	Sets	Reps	Weight	Rest Time	Note

Upper Body

Exercises	Sets	Reps	Weight	1RM	Rest Time	Note

Lower Body

Exercises	Sets	Reps	Weight	1RM	Rest Time	Note

Cool Down

Activity	Sets	Reps	Time	Dist.	Intensity	Note

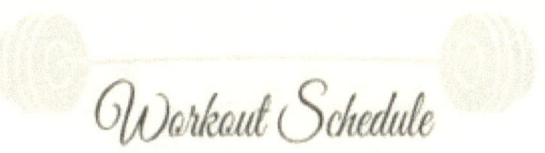

Workout Schedule

Name: _____   Date: _____

Goals: _____

Warm Up

Activity	Sets	Reps	Time	Dist	Intensity	Note

Core Body

Exercises	Sets	Reps	Weight	Rest Time	Note

Upper Body

Exercises	Sets	Reps	Weight	1RM	Rest Time	Note

Lower Body

Exercises	Sets	Reps	Weight	1RM	Rest Time	Note

Cool Down

Activity	Sets	Reps	Time	Dist.	Intensity	Note

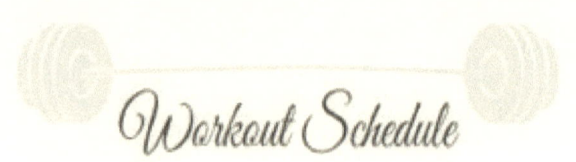

Workout Schedule

Name: _____   Date: _____

Goals: _____

Warm Up

Activity	Sets	Reps	Time	Dist	Intensity	Note

Core Body

Exercises	Sets	Reps	Weight	Rest Time	Note

Upper Body

Exercises	Sets	Reps	Weight	1RM	Rest Time	Note

Lower Body

Exercises	Sets	Reps	Weight	1RM	Rest Time	Note

Cool Down

Activity	Sets	Reps	Time	Dist.	Intensity	Note

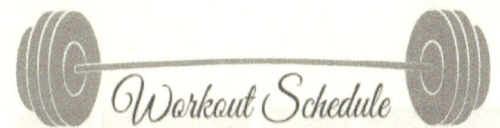

Workout Schedule

NAME: _ _ _ _ _ _ _   DATA: / /

☐ DAY 1

☐ DAY 2

☐ DAY 3

☐ DAY 4

☐ DAY 5

☐ DAY 6

☐ DAY 7

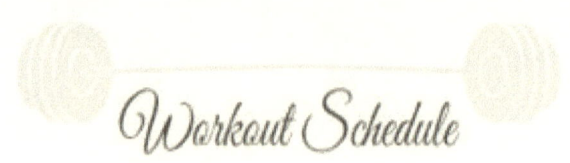

Workout Schedule

Name: _____   Date: _____

Goals: _____

Warm Up

Activity	Sets	Reps	Time	Dist	Intensity	Note

Core Body

Exercises	Sets	Reps	Weight	Rest Time	Note

Upper Body

Exercises	Sets	Reps	Weight	1RM	Rest Time	Note

Lower Body

Exercises	Sets	Reps	Weight	1RM	Rest Time	Note

Cool Down

Activity	Sets	Reps	Time	Dist.	Intensity	Note

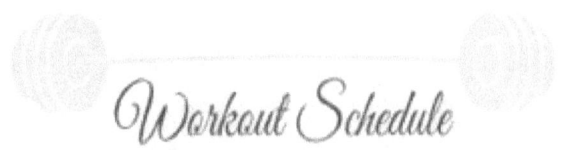

Workout Schedule

Name: Date:

Goals:

Warm Up

Activity	Sets	Reps	Time	Dist	Intensity	Note

Core Body

Exercises	Sets	Reps	Weight	Rest Time	Note

Upper Body

Exercises	Sets	Reps	Weight	1RM	Rest Time	Note

Lower Body

Exercises	Sets	Reps	Weight	1RM	Rest Time	Note

Cool Down

Activity	Sets	Reps	Time	Dist.	Intensity	Note

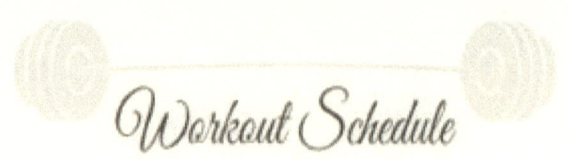

Workout Schedule

Name: _____   Date: _____

Goals: _____

Warm Up

Activity	Sets	Reps	Time	Dist	Intensity	Note

Core Body

Exercises	Sets	Reps	Weight	Rest Time	Note

Upper Body

Exercises	Sets	Reps	Weight	1RM	Rest Time	Note

Lower Body

Exercises	Sets	Reps	Weight	1RM	Rest Time	Note

Cool Down

Activity	Sets	Reps	Time	Dist.	Intensity	Note

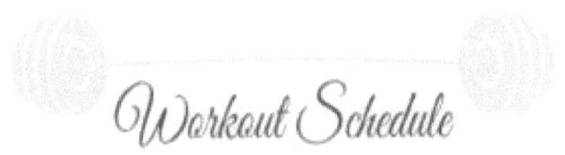

Workout Schedule

Name: Date:

Goals:

Warm Up

Activity	Sets	Reps	Time	Dist	Intensity	Note

Core Body

Exercises	Sets	Reps	Weight	Rest Time	Note

Upper Body

Exercises	Sets	Reps	Weight	1RM	Rest Time	Note

Lower Body

Exercises	Sets	Reps	Weight	1RM	Rest Time	Note

Cool Down

Activity	Sets	Reps	Time	Dist.	Intensity	Note

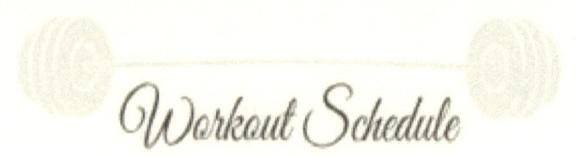

Workout Schedule

Name: _____   Date: _____

Goals: _____

Warm Up

Activity	Sets	Reps	Time	Dist	Intensity	Note

Core Body

Exercises	Sets	Reps	Weight	Rest Time	Note

Upper Body

Exercises	Sets	Reps	Weight	1RM	Rest Time	Note

Lower Body

Exercises	Sets	Reps	Weight	1RM	Rest Time	Note

Cool Down

Activity	Sets	Reps	Time	Dist.	Intensity	Note

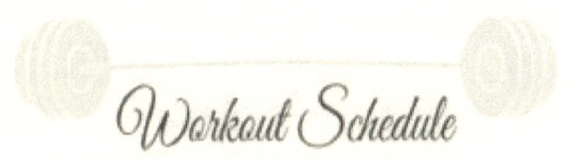

Workout Schedule

Name: _____   Date: _____

Goals: _____

Warm Up

Activity	Sets	Reps	Time	Dist	Intensity	Note

Core Body

Exercises	Sets	Reps	Weight	Rest Time	Note

Upper Body

Exercises	Sets	Reps	Weight	1RM	Rest Time	Note

Lower Body

Exercises	Sets	Reps	Weight	1RM	Rest Time	Note

Cool Down

Activity	Sets	Reps	Time	Dist.	Intensity	Note

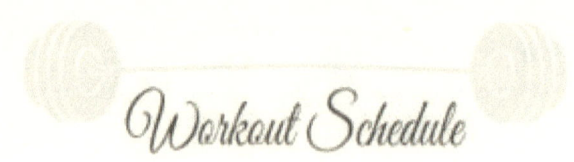

Workout Schedule

Name: Date:

Goals:

Warm Up

Activity	Sets	Reps	Time	Dist	Intensity	Note

Core Body

Exercises	Sets	Reps	Weight	Rest Time	Note

Upper Body

Exercises	Sets	Reps	Weight	1RM	Rest Time	Note

Lower Body

Exercises	Sets	Reps	Weight	1RM	Rest Time	Note

Cool Down

Activity	Sets	Reps	Time	Dist.	Intensity	Note

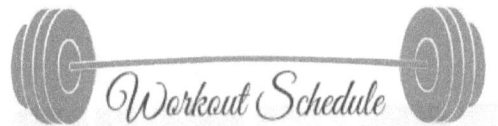

NAME: _ _ _ _ _ _ _   DATA: / /

☐ DAY 1

☐ DAY 2

☐ DAY 3

☐ DAY 4

☐ DAY 5

☐ DAY 6

☐ DAY 7

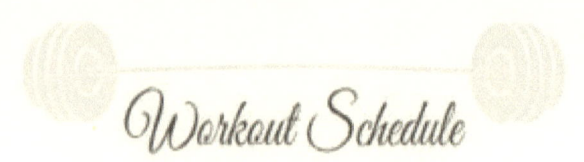

Workout Schedule

Name: _____   Date: _____

Goals: _____

Warm Up

Activity	Sets	Reps	Time	Dist	Intensity	Note

Core Body

Exercises	Sets	Reps	Weight	Rest Time	Note

Upper Body

Exercises	Sets	Reps	Weight	1RM	Rest Time	Note

Lower Body

Exercises	Sets	Reps	Weight	1RM	Rest Time	Note

Cool Down

Activity	Sets	Reps	Time	Dist.	Intensity	Note

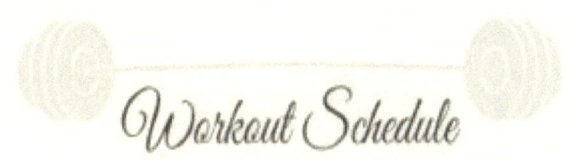

Workout Schedule

Name: _____   Date: _____

Goals: _____

Warm Up

Activity	Sets	Reps	Time	Dist	Intensity	Note

Core Body

Exercises	Sets	Reps	Weight	Rest Time	Note

Upper Body

Exercises	Sets	Reps	Weight	1RM	Rest Time	Note

Lower Body

Exercises	Sets	Reps	Weight	1RM	Rest Time	Note

Cool Down

Activity	Sets	Reps	Time	Dist.	Intensity	Note

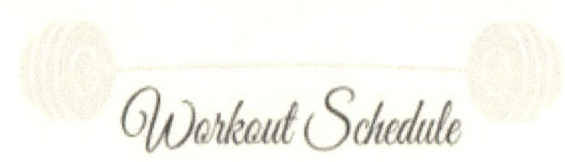

Workout Schedule

Name: _____   Date: _____

Goals: _____

Warm Up

Activity	Sets	Reps	Time	Dist	Intensity	Note

Core Body

Exercises	Sets	Reps	Weight	Rest Time	Note

Upper Body

Exercises	Sets	Reps	Weight	1RM	Rest Time	Note

Lower Body

Exercises	Sets	Reps	Weight	1RM	Rest Time	Note

Cool Down

Activity	Sets	Reps	Time	Dist.	Intensity	Note

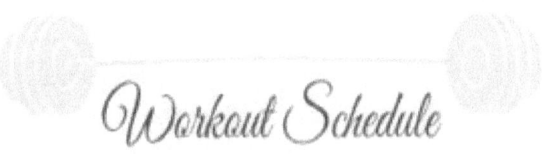

Workout Schedule

Name: Date:

Goals:

Warm Up

Activity	Sets	Reps	Time	Dist	Intensity	Note

Core Body

Exercises	Sets	Reps	Weight	Rest Time	Note

Upper Body

Exercises	Sets	Reps	Weight	1RM	Rest Time	Note

Lower Body

Exercises	Sets	Reps	Weight	1RM	Rest Time	Note

Cool Down

Activity	Sets	Reps	Time	Dist.	Intensity	Note

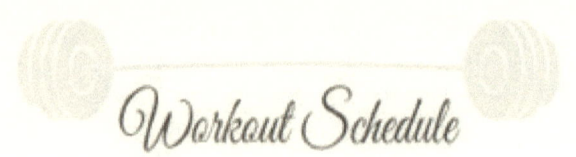

Workout Schedule

Name: _____   Date: _____

Goals: _____

Warm Up

Activity	Sets	Reps	Time	Dist	Intensity	Note

Core Body

Exercises	Sets	Reps	Weight	Rest Time	Note

Upper Body

Exercises	Sets	Reps	Weight	1RM	Rest Time	Note

Lower Body

Exercises	Sets	Reps	Weight	1RM	Rest Time	Note

Cool Down

Activity	Sets	Reps	Time	Dist.	Intensity	Note

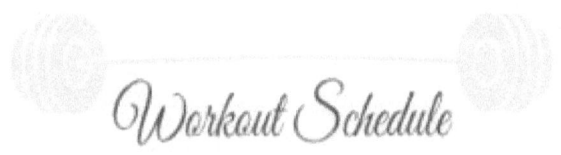

Workout Schedule

Name: Date:

Goals:

Warm Up

Activity	Sets	Reps	Time	Dist	Intensity	Note

Core Body

Exercises	Sets	Reps	Weight	Rest Time	Note

Upper Body

Exercises	Sets	Reps	Weight	1RM	Rest Time	Note

Lower Body

Exercises	Sets	Reps	Weight	1RM	Rest Time	Note

Cool Down

Activity	Sets	Reps	Time	Dist.	Intensity	Note

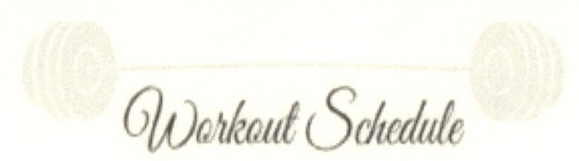

Workout Schedule

Name: _____   Date: _____

Goals: _____

Warm Up

Activity	Sets	Reps	Time	Dist	Intensity	Note

Core Body

Exercises	Sets	Reps	Weight	Rest Time	Note

Upper Body

Exercises	Sets	Reps	Weight	1RM	Rest Time	Note

Lower Body

Exercises	Sets	Reps	Weight	1RM	Rest Time	Note

Cool Down

Activity	Sets	Reps	Time	Dist.	Intensity	Note

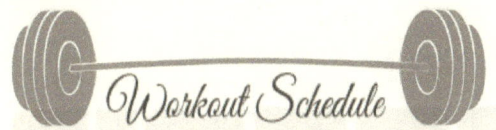

Workout Schedule

NAME: _____   DATA: / /

☐ DAY 1

☐ DAY 2

☐ DAY 3

☐ DAY 4

☐ DAY 5

☐ DAY 6

☐ DAY 7

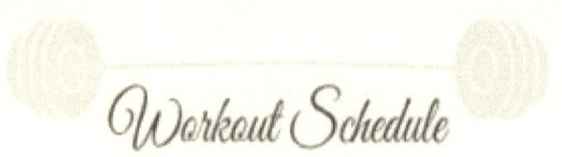

Workout Schedule

Name: _____   Date: _____

Goals: _____

Warm Up

Activity	Sets	Reps	Time	Dist	Intensity	Note

Core Body

Exercises	Sets	Reps	Weight	Rest Time	Note

Upper Body

Exercises	Sets	Reps	Weight	1RM	Rest Time	Note

Lower Body

Exercises	Sets	Reps	Weight	1RM	Rest Time	Note

Cool Down

Activity	Sets	Reps	Time	Dist.	Intensity	Note

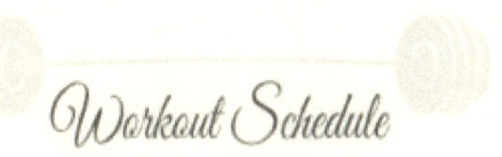

Workout Schedule

Name: _____   Date: _____

Goals: _____

Warm Up

Activity	Sets	Reps	Time	Dist	Intensity	Note

Core Body

Exercises	Sets	Reps	Weight	Rest Time	Note

Upper Body

Exercises	Sets	Reps	Weight	1RM	Rest Time	Note

Lower Body

Exercises	Sets	Reps	Weight	1RM	Rest Time	Note

Cool Down

Activity	Sets	Reps	Time	Dist.	Intensity	Note

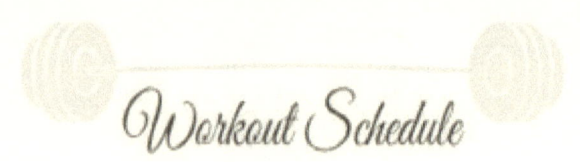

Workout Schedule

Name: _____   Date: _____

Goals: _____

Warm Up

Activity	Sets	Reps	Time	Dist	Intensity	Note

Core Body

Exercises	Sets	Reps	Weight	Rest Time	Note

Upper Body

Exercises	Sets	Reps	Weight	1RM	Rest Time	Note

Lower Body

Exercises	Sets	Reps	Weight	1RM	Rest Time	Note

Cool Down

Activity	Sets	Reps	Time	Dist.	Intensity	Note

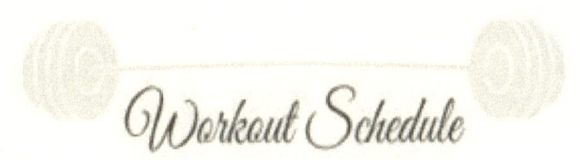

Workout Schedule

Name: _____   Date: _____

Goals: _____

Warm Up

Activity	Sets	Reps	Time	Dist	Intensity	Note

Core Body

Exercises	Sets	Reps	Weight	Rest Time	Note

Upper Body

Exercises	Sets	Reps	Weight	1RM	Rest Time	Note

Lower Body

Exercises	Sets	Reps	Weight	1RM	Rest Time	Note

Cool Down

Activity	Sets	Reps	Time	Dist.	Intensity	Note

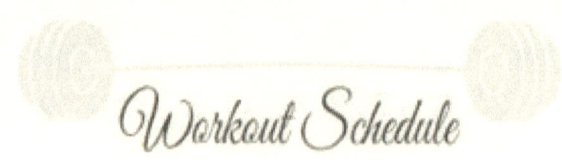

Workout Schedule

Name: _____ Date: _____

Goals: _____

Warm Up

Activity	Sets	Reps	Time	Dist	Intensity	Note

Core Body

Exercises	Sets	Reps	Weight	Rest Time	Note

Upper Body

Exercises	Sets	Reps	Weight	1RM	Rest Time	Note

Lower Body

Exercises	Sets	Reps	Weight	1RM	Rest Time	Note

Cool Down

Activity	Sets	Reps	Time	Dist.	Intensity	Note

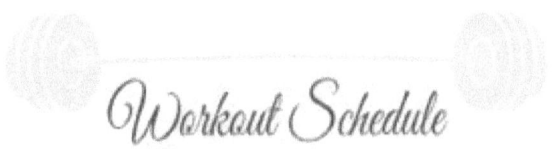

Workout Schedule

Name: _____   Date: _____

Goals: _____

Warm Up

Activity	Sets	Reps	Time	Dist	Intensity	Note

Core Body

Exercises	Sets	Reps	Weight	Rest Time	Note

Upper Body

Exercises	Sets	Reps	Weight	1RM	Rest Time	Note

Lower Body

Exercises	Sets	Reps	Weight	1RM	Rest Time	Note

Cool Down

Activity	Sets	Reps	Time	Dist.	Intensity	Note

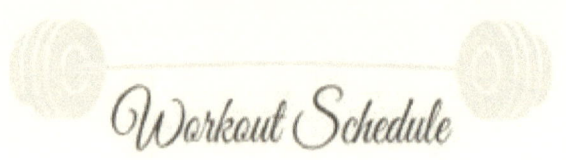

Workout Schedule

Name: _____ Date: _____

Goals: _____

Warm Up

Activity	Sets	Reps	Time	Dist	Intensity	Note

Core Body

Exercises	Sets	Reps	Weight	Rest Time	Note

Upper Body

Exercises	Sets	Reps	Weight	1RM	Rest Time	Note

Lower Body

Exercises	Sets	Reps	Weight	1RM	Rest Time	Note

Cool Down

Activity	Sets	Reps	Time	Dist.	Intensity	Note

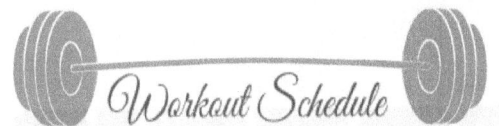

Workout Schedule

NAME: _ _ _ _ _ _ _   DATA: / /

☐ DAY 1

☐ DAY 2

☐ DAY 3

☐ DAY 4

☐ DAY 5

☐ DAY 6

☐ DAY 7

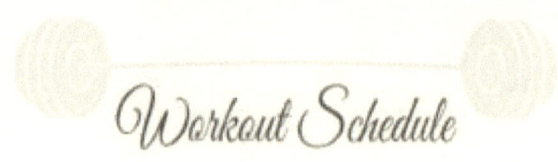

Workout Schedule

Name: _____ **Date:** _____

Goals: _____

Warm Up

Activity	Sets	Reps	Time	Dist	Intensity	Note

Core Body

Exercises	Sets	Reps	Weight	Rest Time	Note

Upper Body

Exercises	Sets	Reps	Weight	1RM	Rest Time	Note

Lower Body

Exercises	Sets	Reps	Weight	1RM	Rest Time	Note

Cool Down

Activity	Sets	Reps	Time	Dist.	Intensity	Note

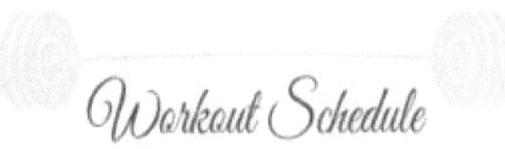

Workout Schedule

Name: Date:

Goals:

Warm Up

Activity	Sets	Reps	Time	Dist	Intensity	Note

Core Body

Exercises	Sets	Reps	Weight	Rest Time	Note

Upper Body

Exercises	Sets	Reps	Weight	1RM	Rest Time	Note

Lower Body

Exercises	Sets	Reps	Weight	1RM	Rest Time	Note

Cool Down

Activity	Sets	Reps	Time	Dist.	Intensity	Note

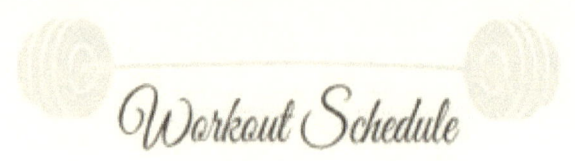

Workout Schedule

Name: _____   Date: _____

Goals: _____

Warm Up

Activity	Sets	Reps	Time	Dist	Intensity	Note

Core Body

Exercises	Sets	Reps	Weight	Rest Time	Note

Upper Body

Exercises	Sets	Reps	Weight	1RM	Rest Time	Note

Lower Body

Exercises	Sets	Reps	Weight	1RM	Rest Time	Note

Cool Down

Activity	Sets	Reps	Time	Dist.	Intensity	Note

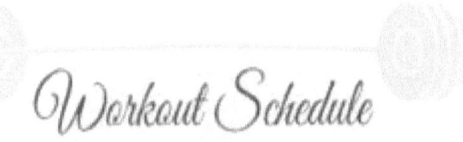

Workout Schedule

Name: Date:

Goals:

Warm Up

Activity	Sets	Reps	Time	Dist	Intensity	Note

Core Body

Exercises	Sets	Reps	Weight	Rest Time	Note

Upper Body

Exercises	Sets	Reps	Weight	1RM	Rest Time	Note

Lower Body

Exercises	Sets	Reps	Weight	1RM	Rest Time	Note

Cool Down

Activity	Sets	Reps	Time	Dist.	Intensity	Note

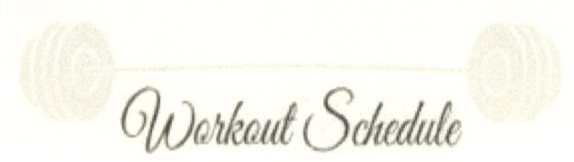

Workout Schedule

Name: _____   Date: _____

Goals: _____

Warm Up

Activity	Sets	Reps	Time	Dist	Intensity	Note

Core Body

Exercises	Sets	Reps	Weight	Rest Time	Note

Upper Body

Exercises	Sets	Reps	Weight	1RM	Rest Time	Note

Lower Body

Exercises	Sets	Reps	Weight	1RM	Rest Time	Note

Cool Down

Activity	Sets	Reps	Time	Dist.	Intensity	Note

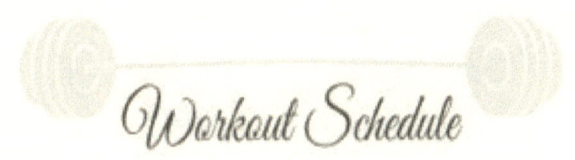

Workout Schedule

Name: _____   Date: _____

Goals: _____

Warm Up

Activity	Sets	Reps	Time	Dist	Intensity	Note

Core Body

Exercises	Sets	Reps	Weight	Rest Time	Note

Upper Body

Exercises	Sets	Reps	Weight	1RM	Rest Time	Note

Lower Body

Exercises	Sets	Reps	Weight	1RM	Rest Time	Note

Cool Down

Activity	Sets	Reps	Time	Dist.	Intensity	Note

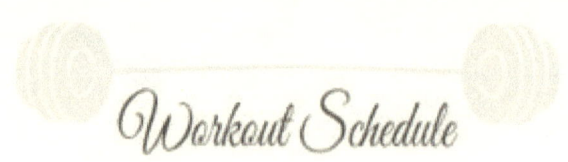

Workout Schedule

Name: _____   Date: _____

Goals: _____

Warm Up

Activity	Sets	Reps	Time	Dist	Intensity	Note

Core Body

Exercises	Sets	Reps	Weight	Rest Time	Note

Upper Body

Exercises	Sets	Reps	Weight	1RM	Rest Time	Note

Lower Body

Exercises	Sets	Reps	Weight	1RM	Rest Time	Note

Cool Down

Activity	Sets	Reps	Time	Dist.	Intensity	Note

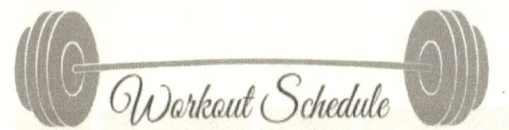

Workout Schedule

NAME: _ _ _ _ _ _ _ _   DATA: / /

☐ DAY 1

☐ DAY 2

☐ DAY 3

☐ DAY 4

☐ DAY 5

☐ DAY 6

☐ DAY 7

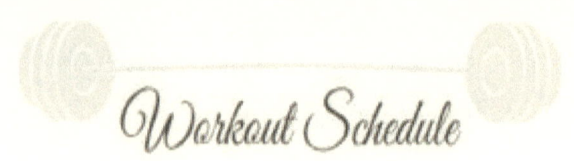

Workout Schedule

Name: Date:

Goals:

Warm Up

Activity	Sets	Reps	Time	Dist	Intensity	Note

Core Body

Exercises	Sets	Reps	Weight	Rest Time	Note

Upper Body

Exercises	Sets	Reps	Weight	1RM	Rest Time	Note

Lower Body

Exercises	Sets	Reps	Weight	1RM	Rest Time	Note

Cool Down

Activity	Sets	Reps	Time	Dist.	Intensity	Note

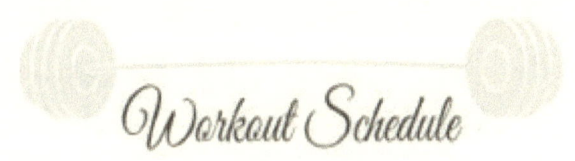

Workout Schedule

Name: _____ Date: _____

Goals: _____

Warm Up

Activity	Sets	Reps	Time	Dist	Intensity	Note

Core Body

Exercises	Sets	Reps	Weight	Rest Time	Note

Upper Body

Exercises	Sets	Reps	Weight	1RM	Rest Time	Note

Lower Body

Exercises	Sets	Reps	Weight	1RM	Rest Time	Note

Cool Down

Activity	Sets	Reps	Time	Dist.	Intensity	Note

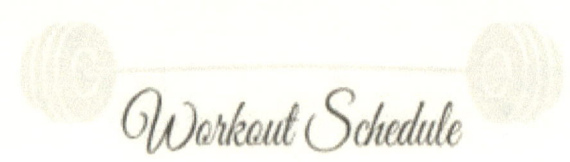

Workout Schedule

Name: _____   Date: _____

Goals: _____

Warm Up

Activity	Sets	Reps	Time	Dist	Intensity	Note

Core Body

Exercises	Sets	Reps	Weight	Rest Time	Note

Upper Body

Exercises	Sets	Reps	Weight	1RM	Rest Time	Note

Lower Body

Exercises	Sets	Reps	Weight	1RM	Rest Time	Note

Cool Down

Activity	Sets	Reps	Time	Dist.	Intensity	Note

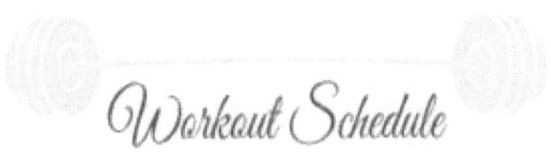

Workout Schedule

Name: Date:

Goals:

Warm Up

Activity	Sets	Reps	Time	Dist	Intensity	Note

Core Body

Exercises	Sets	Reps	Weight	Rest Time	Note

Upper Body

Exercises	Sets	Reps	Weight	1RM	Rest Time	Note

Lower Body

Exercises	Sets	Reps	Weight	1RM	Rest Time	Note

Cool Down

Activity	Sets	Reps	Time	Dist.	Intensity	Note

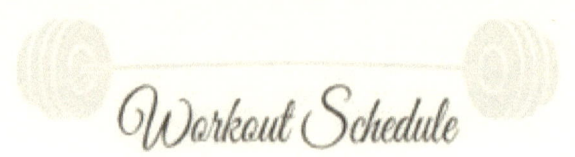

Workout Schedule

Name: _____ Date: _____

Goals: _____

Warm Up

Activity	Sets	Reps	Time	Dist	Intensity	Note

Core Body

Exercises	Sets	Reps	Weight	Rest Time	Note

Upper Body

Exercises	Sets	Reps	Weight	1RM	Rest Time	Note

Lower Body

Exercises	Sets	Reps	Weight	1RM	Rest Time	Note

Cool Down

Activity	Sets	Reps	Time	Dist.	Intensity	Note

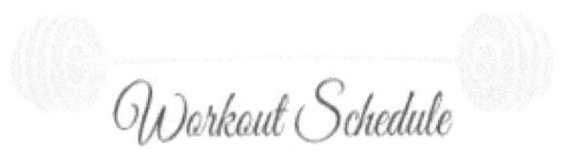

Workout Schedule

Name: Date:

Goals:

Warm Up

Activity	Sets	Reps	Time	Dist	Intensity	Note

Core Body

Exercises	Sets	Reps	Weight	Rest Time	Note

Upper Body

Exercises	Sets	Reps	Weight	1RM	Rest Time	Note

Lower Body

Exercises	Sets	Reps	Weight	1RM	Rest Time	Note

Cool Down

Activity	Sets	Reps	Time	Dist.	Intensity	Note

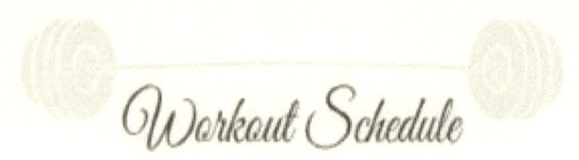

Workout Schedule

Name: Date:

Goals:

Warm Up

Activity	Sets	Reps	Time	Dist	Intensity	Note

Core Body

Exercises	Sets	Reps	Weight	Rest Time	Note

Upper Body

Exercises	Sets	Reps	Weight	1RM	Rest Time	Note

Lower Body

Exercises	Sets	Reps	Weight	1RM	Rest Time	Note

Cool Down

Activity	Sets	Reps	Time	Dist.	Intensity	Note

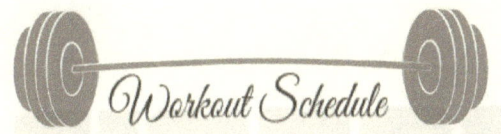

Workout Schedule

NAME: _ _ _ _ _ _ _ _   DATA: / /

☐ DAY 1

☐ DAY 2

☐ DAY 3

☐ DAY 4

☐ DAY 5

☐ DAY 6

☐ DAY 7

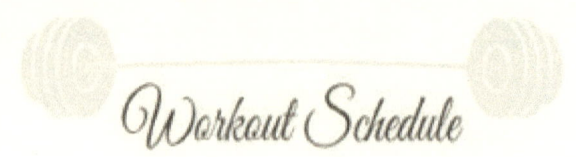

Workout Schedule

Name: _____   Date: _____

Goals: _____

Warm Up

Activity	Sets	Reps	Time	Dist	Intensity	Note

Core Body

Exercises	Sets	Reps	Weight	Rest Time	Note

Upper Body

Exercises	Sets	Reps	Weight	1RM	Rest Time	Note

Lower Body

Exercises	Sets	Reps	Weight	1RM	Rest Time	Note

Cool Down

Activity	Sets	Reps	Time	Dist.	Intensity	Note

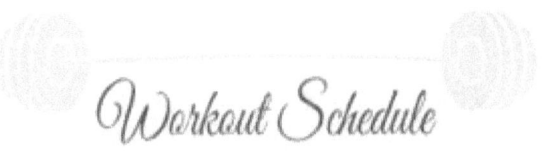

Workout Schedule

Name: Date:

Goals:

Warm Up

Activity	Sets	Reps	Time	Dist	Intensity	Note

Core Body

Exercises	Sets	Reps	Weight	Rest Time	Note

Upper Body

Exercises	Sets	Reps	Weight	1RM	Rest Time	Note

Lower Body

Exercises	Sets	Reps	Weight	1RM	Rest Time	Note

Cool Down

Activity	Sets	Reps	Time	Dist.	Intensity	Note

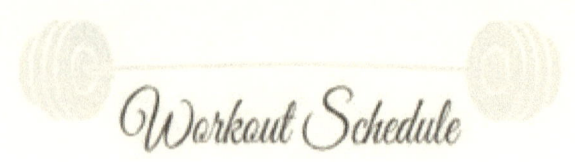

Workout Schedule

Name: _____   Date: _____

Goals: _____

Warm Up

Activity	Sets	Reps	Time	Dist	Intensity	Note

Core Body

Exercises	Sets	Reps	Weight	Rest Time	Note

Upper Body

Exercises	Sets	Reps	Weight	1RM	Rest Time	Note

Lower Body

Exercises	Sets	Reps	Weight	1RM	Rest Time	Note

Cool Down

Activity	Sets	Reps	Time	Dist.	Intensity	Note

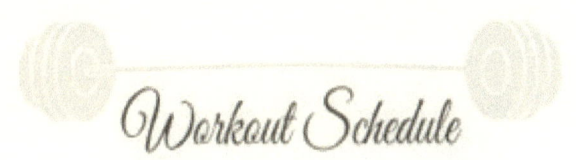

Workout Schedule

Name: _____ Date: _____

Goals: _____

Warm Up

Activity	Sets	Reps	Time	Dist	Intensity	Note

Core Body

Exercises	Sets	Reps	Weight	Rest Time	Note

Upper Body

Exercises	Sets	Reps	Weight	1RM	Rest Time	Note

Lower Body

Exercises	Sets	Reps	Weight	1RM	Rest Time	Note

Cool Down

Activity	Sets	Reps	Time	Dist.	Intensity	Note

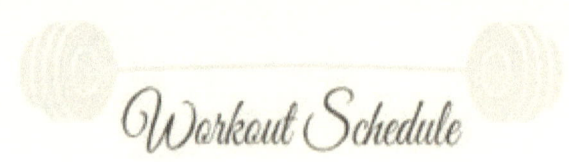

Workout Schedule

Name: _____ Date: _____

Goals: _____

Warm Up

Activity	Sets	Reps	Time	Dist	Intensity	Note

Core Body

Exercises	Sets	Reps	Weight	Rest Time	Note

Upper Body

Exercises	Sets	Reps	Weight	1RM	Rest Time	Note

Lower Body

Exercises	Sets	Reps	Weight	1RM	Rest Time	Note

Cool Down

Activity	Sets	Reps	Time	Dist.	Intensity	Note

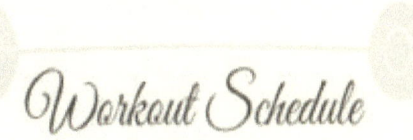

Workout Schedule

Name: _____   Date: _____

Goals: _____

Warm Up

Activity	Sets	Reps	Time	Dist	Intensity	Note

Core Body

Exercises	Sets	Reps	Weight	Rest Time	Note

Upper Body

Exercises	Sets	Reps	Weight	1RM	Rest Time	Note

Lower Body

Exercises	Sets	Reps	Weight	1RM	Rest Time	Note

Cool Down

Activity	Sets	Reps	Time	Dist.	Intensity	Note

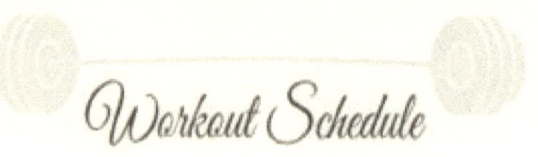

Workout Schedule

Name: Date:

Goals:

Warm Up

Activity	Sets	Reps	Time	Dist	Intensity	Note

Core Body

Exercises	Sets	Reps	Weight	Rest Time	Note

Upper Body

Exercises	Sets	Reps	Weight	1RM	Rest Time	Note

Lower Body

Exercises	Sets	Reps	Weight	1RM	Rest Time	Note

Cool Down

Activity	Sets	Reps	Time	Dist.	Intensity	Note

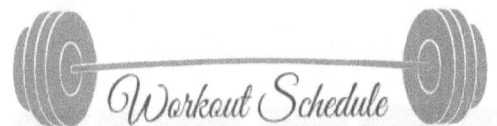

Workout Schedule

NAME: _____

DATA: / /

☐ DAY 1

☐ DAY 2

☐ DAY 3

☐ DAY 4

☐ DAY 5

☐ DAY 6

☐ DAY 7

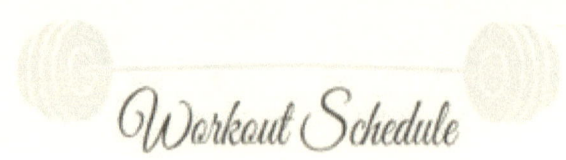

Workout Schedule

Name: _____   Date: _____

Goals: _____

Warm Up

Activity	Sets	Reps	Time	Dist	Intensity	Note

Core Body

Exercises	Sets	Reps	Weight	Rest Time	Note

Upper Body

Exercises	Sets	Reps	Weight	1RM	Rest Time	Note

Lower Body

Exercises	Sets	Reps	Weight	1RM	Rest Time	Note

Cool Down

Activity	Sets	Reps	Time	Dist.	Intensity	Note

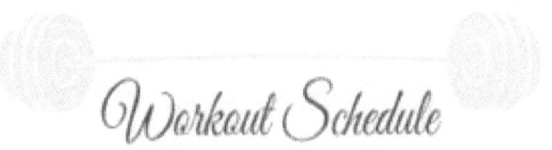

Workout Schedule

Name: _____   Date: _____

Goals: _____

Warm Up

Activity	Sets	Reps	Time	Dist	Intensity	Note

Core Body

Exercises	Sets	Reps	Weight	Rest Time	Note

Upper Body

Exercises	Sets	Reps	Weight	1RM	Rest Time	Note

Lower Body

Exercises	Sets	Reps	Weight	1RM	Rest Time	Note

Cool Down

Activity	Sets	Reps	Time	Dist.	Intensity	Note

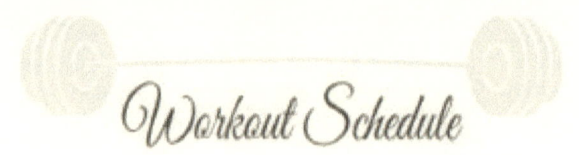

Workout Schedule

Name: _____   **Date:** _____

Goals: _____

Warm Up

Activity	Sets	Reps	Time	Dist	Intensity	Note

Core Body

Exercises	Sets	Reps	Weight	Rest Time	Note

Upper Body

Exercises	Sets	Reps	Weight	1RM	Rest Time	Note

Lower Body

Exercises	Sets	Reps	Weight	1RM	Rest Time	Note

Cool Down

Activity	Sets	Reps	Time	Dist.	Intensity	Note

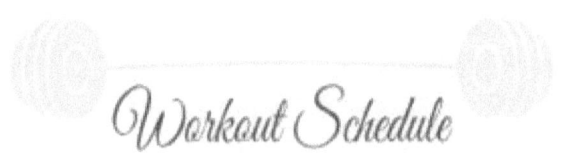

Workout Schedule

Name: Date:

Goals:

Warm Up

Activity	Sets	Reps	Time	Dist	Intensity	Note

Core Body

Exercises	Sets	Reps	Weight	Rest Time	Note

Upper Body

Exercises	Sets	Reps	Weight	1RM	Rest Time	Note

Lower Body

Exercises	Sets	Reps	Weight	1RM	Rest Time	Note

Cool Down

Activity	Sets	Reps	Time	Dist.	Intensity	Note

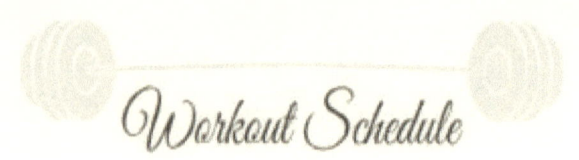

Workout Schedule

Name: _____   Date: _____

Goals: _____

Warm Up

Activity	Sets	Reps	Time	Dist	Intensity	Note

Core Body

Exercises	Sets	Reps	Weight	Rest Time	Note

Upper Body

Exercises	Sets	Reps	Weight	1RM	Rest Time	Note

Lower Body

Exercises	Sets	Reps	Weight	1RM	Rest Time	Note

Cool Down

Activity	Sets	Reps	Time	Dist.	Intensity	Note

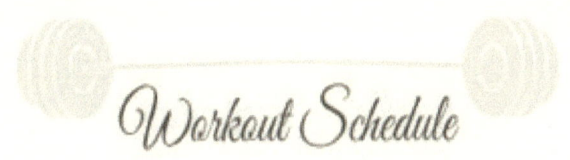

Workout Schedule

Name: _____   Date: _____

Goals: _____

Warm Up

Activity	Sets	Reps	Time	Dist	Intensity	Note

Core Body

Exercises	Sets	Reps	Weight	Rest Time	Note

Upper Body

Exercises	Sets	Reps	Weight	1RM	Rest Time	Note

Lower Body

Exercises	Sets	Reps	Weight	1RM	Rest Time	Note

Cool Down

Activity	Sets	Reps	Time	Dist.	Intensity	Note

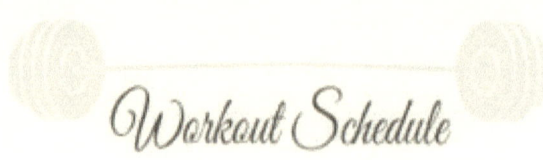

Workout Schedule

Name: _____ Date: _____

Goals: _____

Warm Up

Activity	Sets	Reps	Time	Dist	Intensity	Note

Core Body

Exercises	Sets	Reps	Weight	Rest Time	Note

Upper Body

Exercises	Sets	Reps	Weight	1RM	Rest Time	Note

Lower Body

Exercises	Sets	Reps	Weight	1RM	Rest Time	Note

Cool Down

Activity	Sets	Reps	Time	Dist.	Intensity	Note

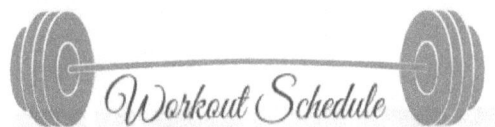

Workout Schedule

NAME: _ _ _ _ _ _ _ _   DATA: / /

☐ DAY 1

☐ DAY 2

☐ DAY 3

☐ DAY 4

☐ DAY 5

☐ DAY 6

☐ DAY 7

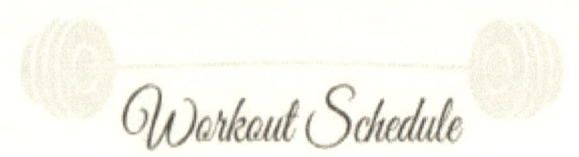

Workout Schedule

Name: _____   Date: _____

Goals: _____

Warm Up

Activity	Sets	Reps	Time	Dist	Intensity	Note

Core Body

Exercises	Sets	Reps	Weight	Rest Time	Note

Upper Body

Exercises	Sets	Reps	Weight	1RM	Rest Time	Note

Lower Body

Exercises	Sets	Reps	Weight	1RM	Rest Time	Note

Cool Down

Activity	Sets	Reps	Time	Dist.	Intensity	Note

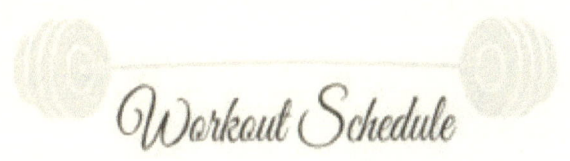

Workout Schedule

Name: _____   Date: _____

Goals: _____

Warm Up

Activity	Sets	Reps	Time	Dist	Intensity	Note

Core Body

Exercises	Sets	Reps	Weight	Rest Time	Note

Upper Body

Exercises	Sets	Reps	Weight	1RM	Rest Time	Note

Lower Body

Exercises	Sets	Reps	Weight	1RM	Rest Time	Note

Cool Down

Activity	Sets	Reps	Time	Dist.	Intensity	Note

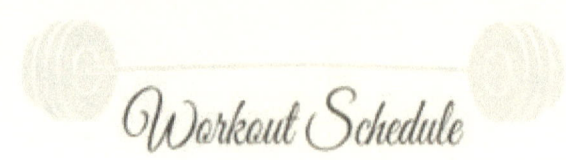

Workout Schedule

Name: _____ Date: _____

Goals: _____

Warm Up

Activity	Sets	Reps	Time	Dist	Intensity	Note

Core Body

Exercises	Sets	Reps	Weight	Rest Time	Note

Upper Body

Exercises	Sets	Reps	Weight	1RM	Rest Time	Note

Lower Body

Exercises	Sets	Reps	Weight	1RM	Rest Time	Note

Cool Down

Activity	Sets	Reps	Time	Dist.	Intensity	Note

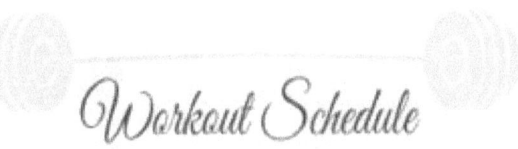

Workout Schedule

Name: _____ Date: _____

Goals: _____

Warm Up

Activity	Sets	Reps	Time	Dist	Intensity	Note

Core Body

Exercises	Sets	Reps	Weight	Rest Time	Note

Upper Body

Exercises	Sets	Reps	Weight	1RM	Rest Time	Note

Lower Body

Exercises	Sets	Reps	Weight	1RM	Rest Time	Note

Cool Down

Activity	Sets	Reps	Time	Dist.	Intensity	Note

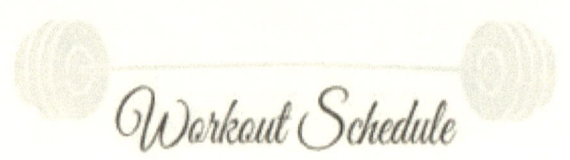

Workout Schedule

Name: _____ Date: _____

Goals: _____

Warm Up

Activity	Sets	Reps	Time	Dist	Intensity	Note

Core Body

Exercises	Sets	Reps	Weight	Rest Time	Note

Upper Body

Exercises	Sets	Reps	Weight	1RM	Rest Time	Note

Lower Body

Exercises	Sets	Reps	Weight	1RM	Rest Time	Note

Cool Down

Activity	Sets	Reps	Time	Dist.	Intensity	Note

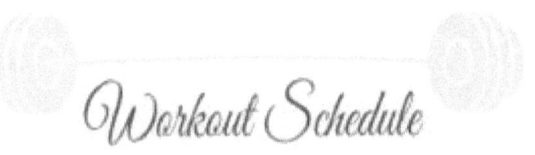

Workout Schedule

Name: Date:

Goals:

Warm Up

Activity	Sets	Reps	Time	Dist	Intensity	Note

Core Body

Exercises	Sets	Reps	Weight	Rest Time	Note

Upper Body

Exercises	Sets	Reps	Weight	1RM	Rest Time	Note

Lower Body

Exercises	Sets	Reps	Weight	1RM	Rest Time	Note

Cool Down

Activity	Sets	Reps	Time	Dist.	Intensity	Note

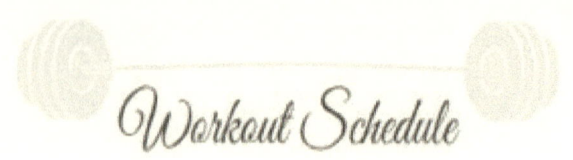

Workout Schedule

Name: _____   Date: _____

Goals: _____

Warm Up

Activity	Sets	Reps	Time	Dist	Intensity	Note

Core Body

Exercises	Sets	Reps	Weight	Rest Time	Note

Upper Body

Exercises	Sets	Reps	Weight	1RM	Rest Time	Note

Lower Body

Exercises	Sets	Reps	Weight	1RM	Rest Time	Note

Cool Down

Activity	Sets	Reps	Time	Dist.	Intensity	Note

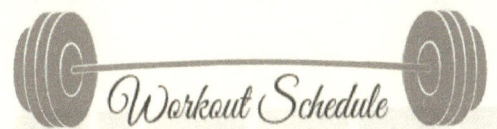

Workout Schedule

NAME: _ _ _ _ _ _ _ _   DATA: / /

☐ DAY 1

☐ DAY 2

☐ DAY 3

☐ DAY 4

☐ DAY 5

☐ DAY 6

☐ DAY 7

NOTES

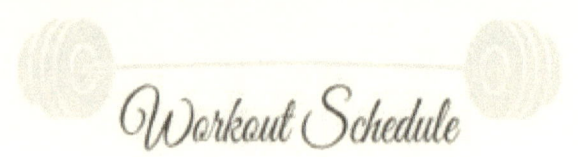

Workout Schedule

Name: _____   Date: _____

Goals: _____

Warm Up

Activity	Sets	Reps	Time	Dist	Intensity	Note

Core Body

Exercises	Sets	Reps	Weight	Rest Time	Note

Upper Body

Exercises	Sets	Reps	Weight	1RM	Rest Time	Note

Lower Body

Exercises	Sets	Reps	Weight	1RM	Rest Time	Note

Cool Down

Activity	Sets	Reps	Time	Dist.	Intensity	Note

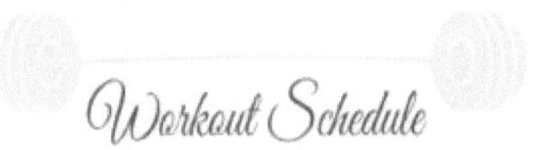

Workout Schedule

Name: Date:

Goals:

Warm Up

Activity	Sets	Reps	Time	Dist	Intensity	Note

Core Body

Exercises	Sets	Reps	Weight	Rest Time	Note

Upper Body

Exercises	Sets	Reps	Weight	1RM	Rest Time	Note

Lower Body

Exercises	Sets	Reps	Weight	1RM	Rest Time	Note

Cool Down

Activity	Sets	Reps	Time	Dist.	Intensity	Note

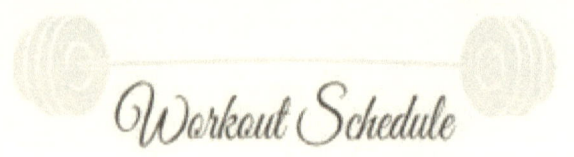

Workout Schedule

Name: _____   Date: _____

Goals: _____

Warm Up

Activity	Sets	Reps	Time	Dist	Intensity	Note

Core Body

Exercises	Sets	Reps	Weight	Rest Time	Note

Upper Body

Exercises	Sets	Reps	Weight	1RM	Rest Time	Note

Lower Body

Exercises	Sets	Reps	Weight	1RM	Rest Time	Note

Cool Down

Activity	Sets	Reps	Time	Dist.	Intensity	Note

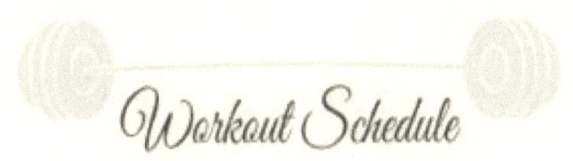

Workout Schedule

Name: _____ Date: _____

Goals: _____

Warm Up

Activity	Sets	Reps	Time	Dist	Intensity	Note

Core Body

Exercises	Sets	Reps	Weight	Rest Time	Note

Upper Body

Exercises	Sets	Reps	Weight	1RM	Rest Time	Note

Lower Body

Exercises	Sets	Reps	Weight	1RM	Rest Time	Note

Cool Down

Activity	Sets	Reps	Time	Dist.	Intensity	Note

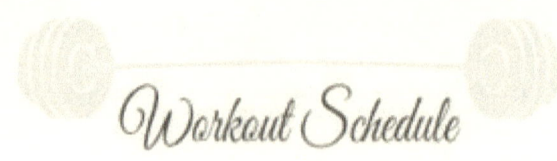

Workout Schedule

Name: _____ Date: _____

Goals: _____

Warm Up

Activity	Sets	Reps	Time	Dist	Intensity	Note

Core Body

Exercises	Sets	Reps	Weight	Rest Time	Note

Upper Body

Exercises	Sets	Reps	Weight	1RM	Rest Time	Note

Lower Body

Exercises	Sets	Reps	Weight	1RM	Rest Time	Note

Cool Down

Activity	Sets	Reps	Time	Dist.	Intensity	Note

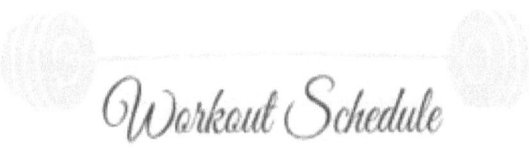

Workout Schedule

Name: Date:

Goals:

Warm Up

Activity	Sets	Reps	Time	Dist	Intensity	Note

Core Body

Exercises	Sets	Reps	Weight	Rest Time	Note

Upper Body

Exercises	Sets	Reps	Weight	1RM	Rest Time	Note

Lower Body

Exercises	Sets	Reps	Weight	1RM	Rest Time	Note

Cool Down

Activity	Sets	Reps	Time	Dist.	Intensity	Note

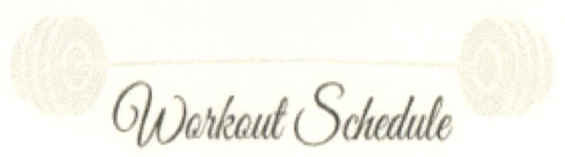

Workout Schedule

Name: _____   Date: _____

Goals: _____

Warm Up

Activity	Sets	Reps	Time	Dist	Intensity	Note

Core Body

Exercises	Sets	Reps	Weight	Rest Time	Note

Upper Body

Exercises	Sets	Reps	Weight	1RM	Rest Time	Note

Lower Body

Exercises	Sets	Reps	Weight	1RM	Rest Time	Note

Cool Down

Activity	Sets	Reps	Time	Dist.	Intensity	Note

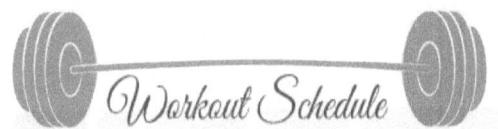

NAME: _ _ _ _ _ _ _

DATA: / /

☐ DAY 1

☐ DAY 2

☐ DAY 3

☐ DAY 4

☐ DAY 5

☐ DAY 6

☐ DAY 7

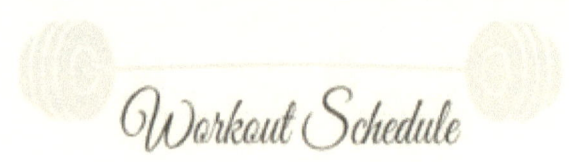

Workout Schedule

Name: _____ Date: _____

Goals: _____

Warm Up

Activity	Sets	Reps	Time	Dist	Intensity	Note

Core Body

Exercises	Sets	Reps	Weight	Rest Time	Note

Upper Body

Exercises	Sets	Reps	Weight	1RM	Rest Time	Note

Lower Body

Exercises	Sets	Reps	Weight	1RM	Rest Time	Note

Cool Down

Activity	Sets	Reps	Time	Dist.	Intensity	Note

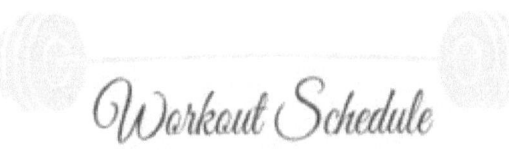

Workout Schedule

Name: Date:

Goals:

Warm Up

Activity	Sets	Reps	Time	Dist	Intensity	Note

Core Body

Exercises	Sets	Reps	Weight	Rest Time	Note

Upper Body

Exercises	Sets	Reps	Weight	1RM	Rest Time	Note

Lower Body

Exercises	Sets	Reps	Weight	1RM	Rest Time	Note

Cool Down

Activity	Sets	Reps	Time	Dist.	Intensity	Note

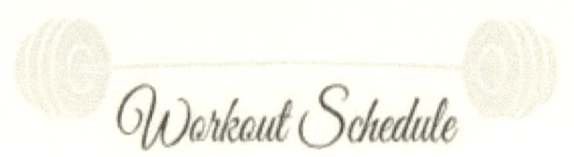

Workout Schedule

Name: _____ Date: _____

Goals: _____

Warm Up

Activity	Sets	Reps	Time	Dist	Intensity	Note

Core Body

Exercises	Sets	Reps	Weight	Rest Time	Note

Upper Body

Exercises	Sets	Reps	Weight	1RM	Rest Time	Note

Lower Body

Exercises	Sets	Reps	Weight	1RM	Rest Time	Note

Cool Down

Activity	Sets	Reps	Time	Dist.	Intensity	Note

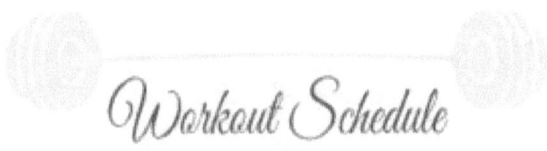

Workout Schedule

Name: Date:

Goals:

Warm Up

Activity	Sets	Reps	Time	Dist	Intensity	Note

Core Body

Exercises	Sets	Reps	Weight	Rest Time	Note

Upper Body

Exercises	Sets	Reps	Weight	1RM	Rest Time	Note

Lower Body

Exercises	Sets	Reps	Weight	1RM	Rest Time	Note

Cool Down

Activity	Sets	Reps	Time	Dist.	Intensity	Note

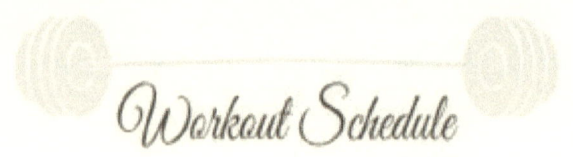

Workout Schedule

Name: _____ Date: _____

Goals: _____

Warm Up

Activity	Sets	Reps	Time	Dist	Intensity	Note

Core Body

Exercises	Sets	Reps	Weight	Rest Time	Note

Upper Body

Exercises	Sets	Reps	Weight	1RM	Rest Time	Note

Lower Body

Exercises	Sets	Reps	Weight	1RM	Rest Time	Note

Cool Down

Activity	Sets	Reps	Time	Dist.	Intensity	Note

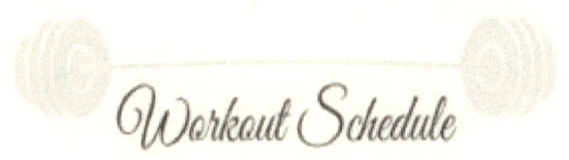

Workout Schedule

Name: _____   Date: _____

Goals: _____

Warm Up

Activity	Sets	Reps	Time	Dist	Intensity	Note

Core Body

Exercises	Sets	Reps	Weight	Rest Time	Note

Upper Body

Exercises	Sets	Reps	Weight	1RM	Rest Time	Note

Lower Body

Exercises	Sets	Reps	Weight	1RM	Rest Time	Note

Cool Down

Activity	Sets	Reps	Time	Dist.	Intensity	Note

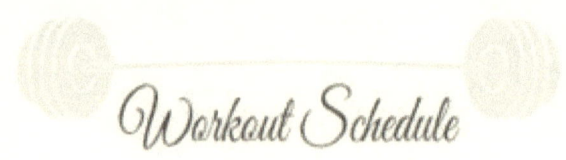

Workout Schedule

Name: _____ Date: _____

Goals: _____

Warm Up

Activity	Sets	Reps	Time	Dist	Intensity	Note

Core Body

Exercises	Sets	Reps	Weight	Rest Time	Note

Upper Body

Exercises	Sets	Reps	Weight	1RM	Rest Time	Note

Lower Body

Exercises	Sets	Reps	Weight	1RM	Rest Time	Note

Cool Down

Activity	Sets	Reps	Time	Dist.	Intensity	Note

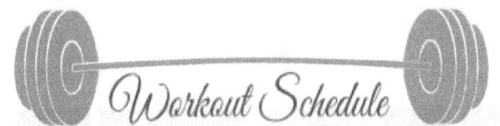

Workout Schedule

NAME: _ _ _ _ _ _ _ _   DATA: / /

☐ DAY 1

☐ DAY 2

☐ DAY 3

☐ DAY 4

☐ DAY 5

☐ DAY 6

☐ DAY 7

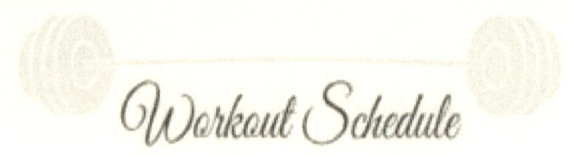

Workout Schedule

Name: _____   Date: _____

Goals: _____

Warm Up

Activity	Sets	Reps	Time	Dist	Intensity	Note

Core Body

Exercises	Sets	Reps	Weight	Rest Time	Note

Upper Body

Exercises	Sets	Reps	Weight	1RM	Rest Time	Note

Lower Body

Exercises	Sets	Reps	Weight	1RM	Rest Time	Note

Cool Down

Activity	Sets	Reps	Time	Dist.	Intensity	Note

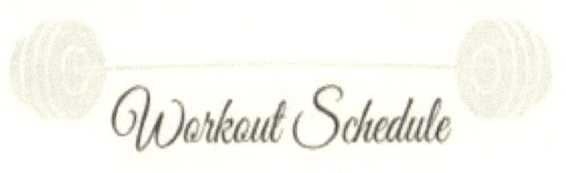

Workout Schedule

Name: _____   Date: _____

Goals: _____

Warm Up

Activity	Sets	Reps	Time	Dist	Intensity	Note

Core Body

Exercises	Sets	Reps	Weight	Rest Time	Note

Upper Body

Exercises	Sets	Reps	Weight	1RM	Rest Time	Note

Lower Body

Exercises	Sets	Reps	Weight	1RM	Rest Time	Note

Cool Down

Activity	Sets	Reps	Time	Dist.	Intensity	Note

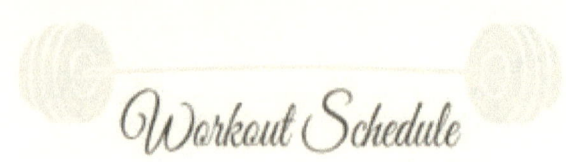

Workout Schedule

Name: _____   Date: _____

Goals: _____

Warm Up

Activity	Sets	Reps	Time	Dist	Intensity	Note

Core Body

Exercises	Sets	Reps	Weight	Rest Time	Note

Upper Body

Exercises	Sets	Reps	Weight	1RM	Rest Time	Note

Lower Body

Exercises	Sets	Reps	Weight	1RM	Rest Time	Note

Cool Down

Activity	Sets	Reps	Time	Dist.	Intensity	Note

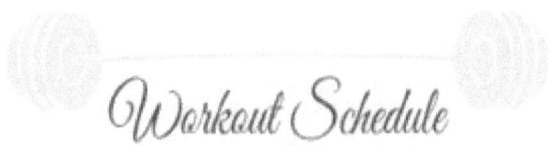

Workout Schedule

Name: Date:

Goals:

Warm Up

Activity	Sets	Reps	Time	Dist	Intensity	Note

Core Body

Exercises	Sets	Reps	Weight	Rest Time	Note

Upper Body

Exercises	Sets	Reps	Weight	1RM	Rest Time	Note

Lower Body

Exercises	Sets	Reps	Weight	1RM	Rest Time	Note

Cool Down

Activity	Sets	Reps	Time	Dist.	Intensity	Note

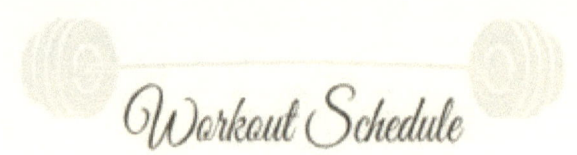

Workout Schedule

Name: _____   Date: _____

Goals: _____

Warm Up

Activity	Sets	Reps	Time	Dist	Intensity	Note

Core Body

Exercises	Sets	Reps	Weight	Rest Time	Note

Upper Body

Exercises	Sets	Reps	Weight	1RM	Rest Time	Note

Lower Body

Exercises	Sets	Reps	Weight	1RM	Rest Time	Note

Cool Down

Activity	Sets	Reps	Time	Dist.	Intensity	Note

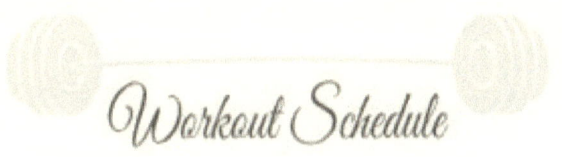

Workout Schedule

Name: _____   Date: _____

Goals: _____

Warm Up

Activity	Sets	Reps	Time	Dist	Intensity	Note

Core Body

Exercises	Sets	Reps	Weight	Rest Time	Note

Upper Body

Exercises	Sets	Reps	Weight	1RM	Rest Time	Note

Lower Body

Exercises	Sets	Reps	Weight	1RM	Rest Time	Note

Cool Down

Activity	Sets	Reps	Time	Dist.	Intensity	Note

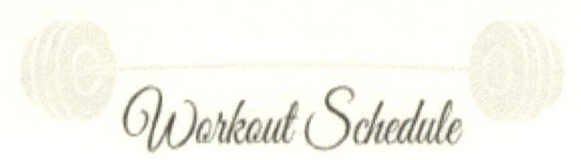

Workout Schedule

Name: _____   Date: _____

Goals: _____

Warm Up

Activity	Sets	Reps	Time	Dist	Intensity	Note

Core Body

Exercises	Sets	Reps	Weight	Rest Time	Note

Upper Body

Exercises	Sets	Reps	Weight	1RM	Rest Time	Note

Lower Body

Exercises	Sets	Reps	Weight	1RM	Rest Time	Note

Cool Down

Activity	Sets	Reps	Time	Dist.	Intensity	Note

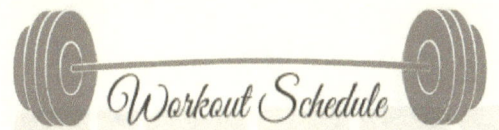

Workout Schedule

NAME: _____   DATA: / /

☐ DAY 1

☐ DAY 2

☐ DAY 3

☐ DAY 4

☐ DAY 5

☐ DAY 6

☐ DAY 7

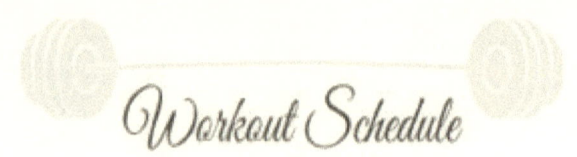

Workout Schedule

Name: _____   Date: _____

Goals: _____

Warm Up

	Activity	Sets	Reps	Time	Dist	Intensity	Note

Core Body

	Exercises	Sets	Reps	Weight	Rest Time	Note

Upper Body

	Exercises	Sets	Reps	Weight	1RM	Rest Time	Note

Lower Body

	Exercises	Sets	Reps	Weight	1RM	Rest Time	Note

Cool Down

	Activity	Sets	Reps	Time	Dist.	Intensity	Note

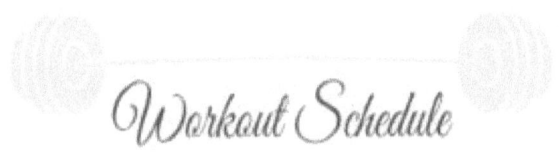

Workout Schedule

Name: Date:

Goals:

Warm Up

Activity	Sets	Reps	Time	Dist	Intensity	Note

Core Body

Exercises	Sets	Reps	Weight	Rest Time	Note

Upper Body

Exercises	Sets	Reps	Weight	1RM	Rest Time	Note

Lower Body

Exercises	Sets	Reps	Weight	1RM	Rest Time	Note

Cool Down

Activity	Sets	Reps	Time	Dist.	Intensity	Note

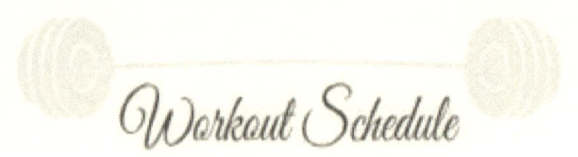

Workout Schedule

Name: _____ Date: _____

Goals: _____

Warm Up

Activity	Sets	Reps	Time	Dist	Intensity	Note

Core Body

Exercises	Sets	Reps	Weight	Rest Time	Note

Upper Body

Exercises	Sets	Reps	Weight	1RM	Rest Time	Note

Lower Body

Exercises	Sets	Reps	Weight	1RM	Rest Time	Note

Cool Down

Activity	Sets	Reps	Time	Dist.	Intensity	Note

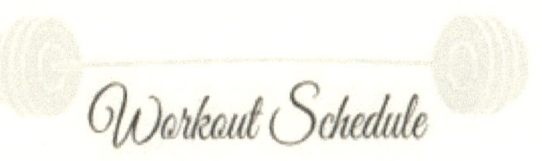

Workout Schedule

Name: _____   Date: _____

Goals: _____

Warm Up

Activity	Sets	Reps	Time	Dist	Intensity	Note

Core Body

Exercises	Sets	Reps	Weight	Rest Time	Note

Upper Body

Exercises	Sets	Reps	Weight	1RM	Rest Time	Note

Lower Body

Exercises	Sets	Reps	Weight	1RM	Rest Time	Note

Cool Down

Activity	Sets	Reps	Time	Dist.	Intensity	Note

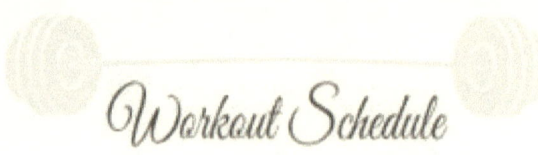

Workout Schedule

Name: _____   Date: _____

Goals: _____

Warm Up

Activity	Sets	Reps	Time	Dist	Intensity	Note

Core Body

Exercises	Sets	Reps	Weight	Rest Time	Note

Upper Body

Exercises	Sets	Reps	Weight	1RM	Rest Time	Note

Lower Body

Exercises	Sets	Reps	Weight	1RM	Rest Time	Note

Cool Down

Activity	Sets	Reps	Time	Dist.	Intensity	Note

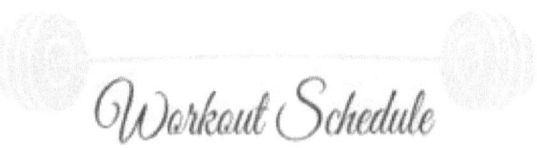

Workout Schedule

Name: Date:

Goals:

Warm Up

Activity	Sets	Reps	Time	Dist	Intensity	Note

Core Body

Exercises	Sets	Reps	Weight	Rest Time	Note

Upper Body

Exercises	Sets	Reps	Weight	1RM	Rest Time	Note

Lower Body

Exercises	Sets	Reps	Weight	1RM	Rest Time	Note

Cool Down

Activity	Sets	Reps	Time	Dist.	Intensity	Note

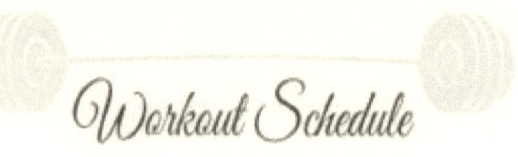

Workout Schedule

Name: _____ **Date:** _____

Goals: _____

Warm Up

Activity	Sets	Reps	Time	Dist	Intensity	Note

Core Body

Exercises	Sets	Reps	Weight	Rest Time	Note

Upper Body

Exercises	Sets	Reps	Weight	1RM	Rest Time	Note

Lower Body

Exercises	Sets	Reps	Weight	1RM	Rest Time	Note

Cool Down

Activity	Sets	Reps	Time	Dist.	Intensity	Note

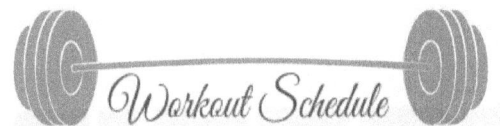

NAME: _ _ _ _ _ _ _ _

DATA: / /

☐ DAY 1

☐ DAY 2

☐ DAY 3

☐ DAY 4

☐ DAY 5

☐ DAY 6

☐ DAY 7

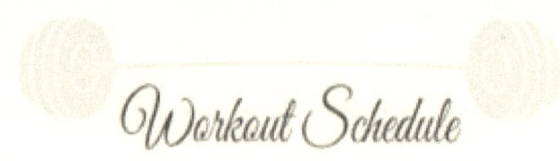

Workout Schedule

Name: _____   Date: _____

Goals: _____

Warm Up

Activity	Sets	Reps	Time	Dist	Intensity	Note

Core Body

Exercises	Sets	Reps	Weight	Rest Time	Note

Upper Body

Exercises	Sets	Reps	Weight	1RM	Rest Time	Note

Lower Body

Exercises	Sets	Reps	Weight	1RM	Rest Time	Note

Cool Down

Activity	Sets	Reps	Time	Dist.	Intensity	Note

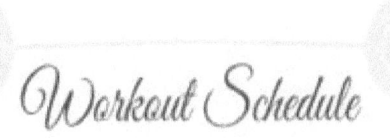

Workout Schedule

Name: _____   Date: _____

Goals: _____

Warm Up

Activity	Sets	Reps	Time	Dist	Intensity	Note

Core Body

Exercises	Sets	Reps	Weight	Rest Time	Note

Upper Body

Exercises	Sets	Reps	Weight	1RM	Rest Time	Note

Lower Body

Exercises	Sets	Reps	Weight	1RM	Rest Time	Note

Cool Down

Activity	Sets	Reps	Time	Dist.	Intensity	Note

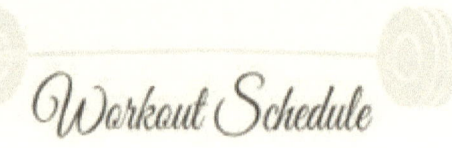

Workout Schedule

Name: _____   Date: _____

Goals: _____

Warm Up

Activity	Sets	Reps	Time	Dist	Intensity	Note

Core Body

Exercises	Sets	Reps	Weight	Rest Time		Note

Upper Body

Exercises	Sets	Reps	Weight	1RM	Rest Time	Note

Lower Body

Exercises	Sets	Reps	Weight	1RM	Rest Time	Note

Cool Down

Activity	Sets	Reps	Time	Dist.	Intensity	Note

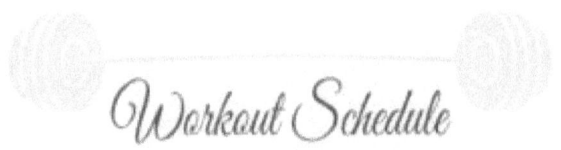

Workout Schedule

Name: Date:

Goals:

Warm Up

Activity	Sets	Reps	Time	Dist	Intensity	Note

Core Body

Exercises	Sets	Reps	Weight	Rest Time	Note

Upper Body

Exercises	Sets	Reps	Weight	1RM	Rest Time	Note

Lower Body

Exercises	Sets	Reps	Weight	1RM	Rest Time	Note

Cool Down

Activity	Sets	Reps	Time	Dist.	Intensity	Note

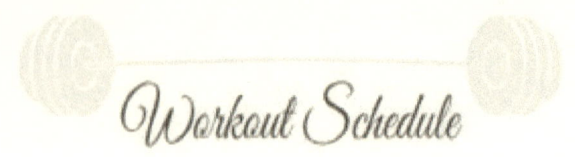

Workout Schedule

Name: _____   Date: _____

Goals: _____

Warm Up

Activity	Sets	Reps	Time	Dist	Intensity	Note

Core Body

Exercises	Sets	Reps	Weight	Rest Time	Note

Upper Body

Exercises	Sets	Reps	Weight	1RM	Rest Time	Note

Lower Body

Exercises	Sets	Reps	Weight	1RM	Rest Time	Note

Cool Down

Activity	Sets	Reps	Time	Dist.	Intensity	Note

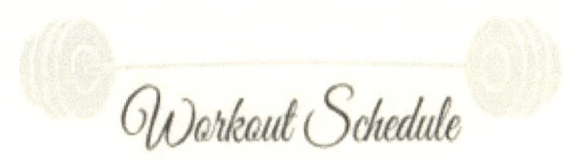

Workout Schedule

Name: _____ **Date:** _____

Goals: _____

Warm Up

Activity	Sets	Reps	Time	Dist	Intensity	Note

Core Body

Exercises	Sets	Reps	Weight	Rest Time	Note

Upper Body

Exercises	Sets	Reps	Weight	1RM	Rest Time	Note

Lower Body

Exercises	Sets	Reps	Weight	1RM	Rest Time	Note

Cool Down

Activity	Sets	Reps	Time	Dist.	Intensity	Note

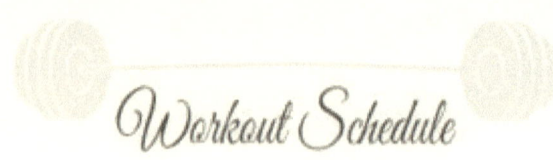

Workout Schedule

Name: _____   Date: _____

Goals: _____

Warm Up

Activity	Sets	Reps	Time	Dist	Intensity	Note

Core Body

Exercises	Sets	Reps	Weight	Rest Time	Note

Upper Body

Exercises	Sets	Reps	Weight	1RM	Rest Time	Note

Lower Body

Exercises	Sets	Reps	Weight	1RM	Rest Time	Note

Cool Down

Activity	Sets	Reps	Time	Dist.	Intensity	Note

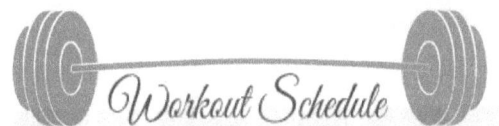

Workout Schedule

NAME: _ _ _ _ _ _ _

DATA: / /

☐ DAY 1

☐ DAY 2

☐ DAY 3

☐ DAY 4

☐ DAY 5

☐ DAY 6

☐ DAY 7

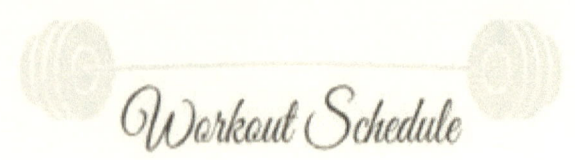

Workout Schedule

Name: _____   Date: _____

Goals: _____

Warm Up

Activity	Sets	Reps	Time	Dist	Intensity	Note

Core Body

Exercises	Sets	Reps	Weight	Rest Time	Note

Upper Body

Exercises	Sets	Reps	Weight	1RM	Rest Time	Note

Lower Body

Exercises	Sets	Reps	Weight	1RM	Rest Time	Note

Cool Down

Activity	Sets	Reps	Time	Dist.	Intensity	Note

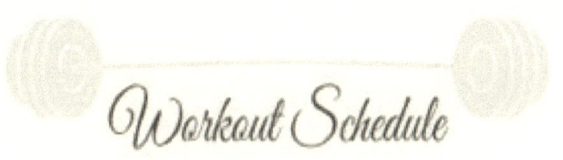

Workout Schedule

Name: _____   Date: _____

Goals: _____

Warm Up

Activity	Sets	Reps	Time	Dist	Intensity	Note

Core Body

Exercises	Sets	Reps	Weight	Rest Time	Note

Upper Body

Exercises	Sets	Reps	Weight	1RM	Rest Time	Note

Lower Body

Exercises	Sets	Reps	Weight	1RM	Rest Time	Note

Cool Down

Activity	Sets	Reps	Time	Dist.	Intensity	Note

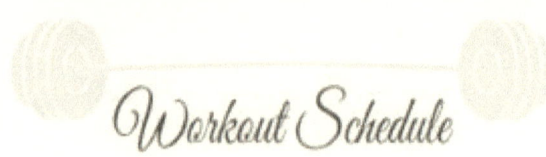

Workout Schedule

Name: _____   Date: _____

Goals: _____

Warm Up

Activity	Sets	Reps	Time	Dist	Intensity	Note

Core Body

Exercises	Sets	Reps	Weight	Rest Time	Note

Upper Body

Exercises	Sets	Reps	Weight	1RM	Rest Time	Note

Lower Body

Exercises	Sets	Reps	Weight	1RM	Rest Time	Note

Cool Down

Activity	Sets	Reps	Time	Dist.	Intensity	Note

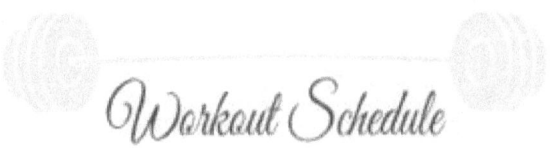

Workout Schedule

Name: _____   Date: _____

Goals: _____

Warm Up

Activity	Sets	Reps	Time	Dist	Intensity	Note

Core Body

Exercises	Sets	Reps	Weight	Rest Time	Note

Upper Body

Exercises	Sets	Reps	Weight	1RM	Rest Time	Note

Lower Body

Exercises	Sets	Reps	Weight	1RM	Rest Time	Note

Cool Down

Activity	Sets	Reps	Time	Dist.	Intensity	Note

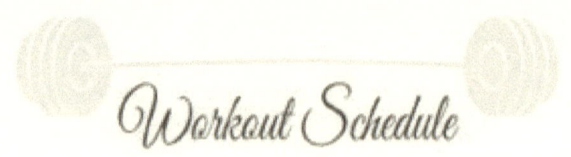

Workout Schedule

Name: _____ Date: _____

Goals: _____

Warm Up

Activity	Sets	Reps	Time	Dist	Intensity	Note

Core Body

Exercises	Sets	Reps	Weight	Rest Time	Note

Upper Body

Exercises	Sets	Reps	Weight	1RM	Rest Time	Note

Lower Body

Exercises	Sets	Reps	Weight	1RM	Rest Time	Note

Cool Down

Activity	Sets	Reps	Time	Dist.	Intensity	Note

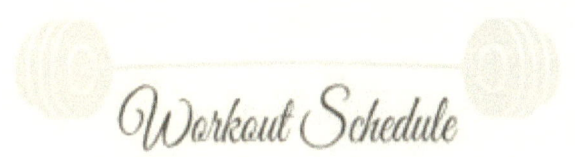

Workout Schedule

Name: **Date:**

Goals:

Warm Up

Activity	Sets	Reps	Time	Dist	Intensity	Note

Core Body

Exercises	Sets	Reps	Weight	Rest Time	Note

Upper Body

Exercises	Sets	Reps	Weight	1RM	Rest Time	Note

Lower Body

Exercises	Sets	Reps	Weight	1RM	Rest Time	Note

Cool Down

Activity	Sets	Reps	Time	Dist.	Intensity	Note

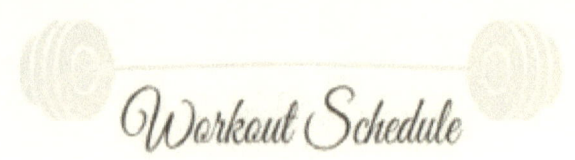

Workout Schedule

Name: _____   Date: _____

Goals: _____

Warm Up

Activity	Sets	Reps	Time	Dist	Intensity	Note

Core Body

Exercises	Sets	Reps	Weight	Rest Time	Note

Upper Body

Exercises	Sets	Reps	Weight	1RM	Rest Time	Note

Lower Body

Exercises	Sets	Reps	Weight	1RM	Rest Time	Note

Cool Down

Activity	Sets	Reps	Time	Dist.	Intensity	Note

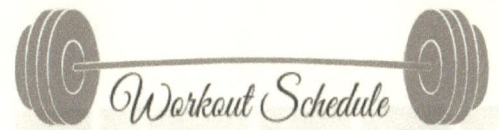

Workout Schedule

NAME: _ _ _ _ _ _ _   DATA: / /

☐ DAY 1

☐ DAY 2

☐ DAY 3

☐ DAY 4

☐ DAY 5

☐ DAY 6

☐ DAY 7

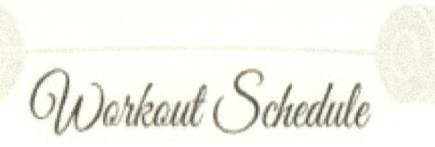

Workout Schedule

Name: _____   Date: _____

Goals: _____

Warm Up

Activity	Sets	Reps	Time	Dist	Intensity	Note

Core Body

Exercises	Sets	Reps	Weight	Rest Time	Note

Upper Body

Exercises	Sets	Reps	Weight	1RM	Rest Time	Note

Lower Body

Exercises	Sets	Reps	Weight	1RM	Rest Time	Note

Cool Down

Activity	Sets	Reps	Time	Dist.	Intensity	Note

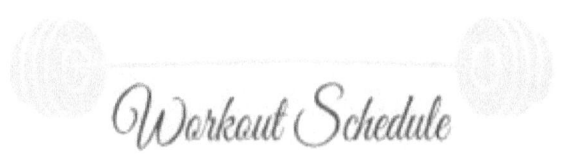

Workout Schedule

Name: Date:

Goals:

Warm Up

Activity	Sets	Reps	Time	Dist	Intensity	Note

Core Body

Exercises	Sets	Reps	Weight	Rest Time	Note

Upper Body

Exercises	Sets	Reps	Weight	1RM	Rest Time	Note

Lower Body

Exercises	Sets	Reps	Weight	1RM	Rest Time	Note

Cool Down

Activity	Sets	Reps	Time	Dist.	Intensity	Note

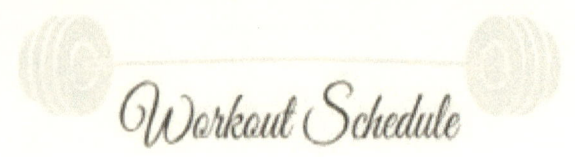

Workout Schedule

Name: _____   Date: _____

Goals: _____

Warm Up

Activity	Sets	Reps	Time	Dist	Intensity	Note

Core Body

Exercises	Sets	Reps	Weight	Rest Time	Note

Upper Body

Exercises	Sets	Reps	Weight	1RM	Rest Time	Note

Lower Body

Exercises	Sets	Reps	Weight	1RM	Rest Time	Note

Cool Down

Activity	Sets	Reps	Time	Dist.	Intensity	Note

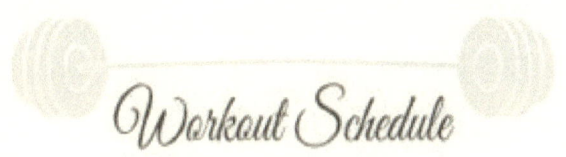

Workout Schedule

Name: _____ Date: _____

Goals: _____

Warm Up

Activity	Sets	Reps	Time	Dist	Intensity	Note

Core Body

Exercises	Sets	Reps	Weight	Rest Time	Note

Upper Body

Exercises	Sets	Reps	Weight	1RM	Rest Time	Note

Lower Body

Exercises	Sets	Reps	Weight	1RM	Rest Time	Note

Cool Down

Activity	Sets	Reps	Time	Dist.	Intensity	Note

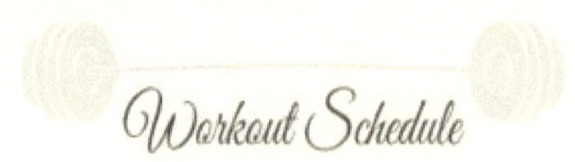

Workout Schedule

Name: _____   Date: _____

Goals: _____

Warm Up

Activity	Sets	Reps	Time	Dist	Intensity	Note

Core Body

Exercises	Sets	Reps	Weight	Rest Time	Note

Upper Body

Exercises	Sets	Reps	Weight	1RM	Rest Time	Note

Lower Body

Exercises	Sets	Reps	Weight	1RM	Rest Time	Note

Cool Down

Activity	Sets	Reps	Time	Dist.	Intensity	Note

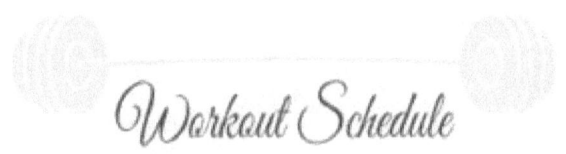

Workout Schedule

Name: Date:

Goals:

Warm Up

Activity	Sets	Reps	Time	Dist	Intensity	Note

Core Body

Exercises	Sets	Reps	Weight	Rest Time	Note

Upper Body

Exercises	Sets	Reps	Weight	1RM	Rest Time	Note

Lower Body

Exercises	Sets	Reps	Weight	1RM	Rest Time	Note

Cool Down

Activity	Sets	Reps	Time	Dist.	Intensity	Note

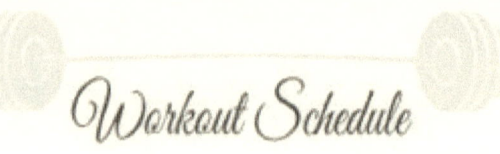

Workout Schedule

Name: _____ Date: _____

Goals: _____

Warm Up

Activity	Sets	Reps	Time	Dist	Intensity	Note

Core Body

Exercises	Sets	Reps	Weight	Rest Time	Note

Upper Body

Exercises	Sets	Reps	Weight	1RM	Rest Time	Note

Lower Body

Exercises	Sets	Reps	Weight	1RM	Rest Time	Note

Cool Down

Activity	Sets	Reps	Time	Dist.	Intensity	Note

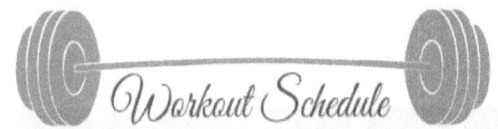

Workout Schedule

NAME: _ _ _ _ _ _ _

DATA: / /

☐ DAY 1

☐ DAY 2

☐ DAY 3

☐ DAY 4

☐ DAY 5

☐ DAY 6

☐ DAY 7

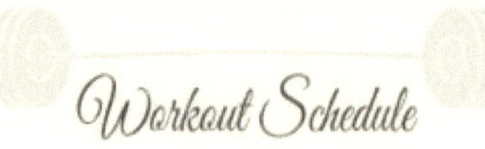

Workout Schedule

Name: _____ Date: _____

Goals: _____

Warm Up

Activity	Sets	Reps	Time	Dist	Intensity	Note

Core Body

Exercises	Sets	Reps	Weight	Rest Time	Note

Upper Body

Exercises	Sets	Reps	Weight	1RM	Rest Time	Note

Lower Body

Exercises	Sets	Reps	Weight	1RM	Rest Time	Note

Cool Down

Activity	Sets	Reps	Time	Dist.	Intensity	Note

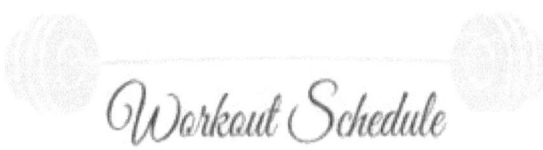

Workout Schedule

Name: Date:

Goals:

Warm Up

Activity	Sets	Reps	Time	Dist	Intensity	Note

Core Body

Exercises	Sets	Reps	Weight	Rest Time	Note

Upper Body

Exercises	Sets	Reps	Weight	1RM	Rest Time	Note

Lower Body

Exercises	Sets	Reps	Weight	1RM	Rest Time	Note

Cool Down

Activity	Sets	Reps	Time	Dist.	Intensity	Note

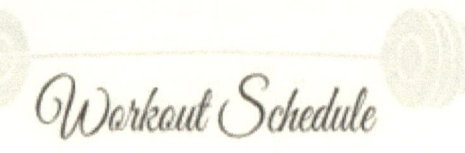

Workout Schedule

Name: _____   Date: _____

Goals: _____

Warm Up

Activity	Sets	Reps	Time	Dist	Intensity	Note

Core Body

Exercises	Sets	Reps	Weight	Rest Time	Note

Upper Body

Exercises	Sets	Reps	Weight	1RM	Rest Time	Note

Lower Body

Exercises	Sets	Reps	Weight	1RM	Rest Time	Note

Cool Down

Activity	Sets	Reps	Time	Dist.	Intensity	Note

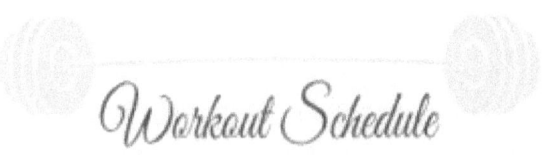

Workout Schedule

Name: Date:

Goals:

Warm Up

Activity	Sets	Reps	Time	Dist	Intensity	Note

Core Body

Exercises	Sets	Reps	Weight	Rest Time	Note

Upper Body

Exercises	Sets	Reps	Weight	1RM	Rest Time	Note

Lower Body

Exercises	Sets	Reps	Weight	1RM	Rest Time	Note

Cool Down

Activity	Sets	Reps	Time	Dist.	Intensity	Note

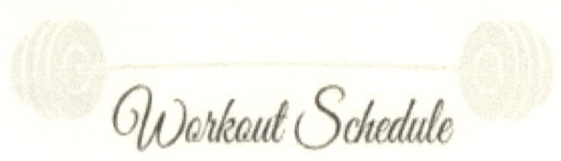

Workout Schedule

Name: _____   Date: _____

Goals: _____

Warm Up

Activity	Sets	Reps	Time	Dist	Intensity	Note

Core Body

Exercises	Sets	Reps	Weight	Rest Time	Note

Upper Body

Exercises	Sets	Reps	Weight	1RM	Rest Time	Note

Lower Body

Exercises	Sets	Reps	Weight	1RM	Rest Time	Note

Cool Down

Activity	Sets	Reps	Time	Dist.	Intensity	Note

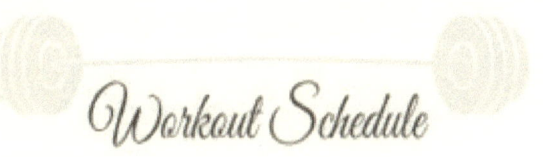

Workout Schedule

Name: _____   Date: _____

Goals: _____

Warm Up

Activity	Sets	Reps	Time	Dist	Intensity	Note

Core Body

Exercises	Sets	Reps	Weight	Rest Time	Note

Upper Body

Exercises	Sets	Reps	Weight	1RM	Rest Time	Note

Lower Body

Exercises	Sets	Reps	Weight	1RM	Rest Time	Note

Cool Down

Activity	Sets	Reps	Time	Dist.	Intensity	Note

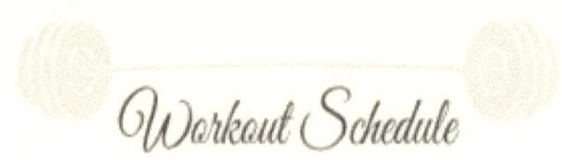

Workout Schedule

Name: _____ Date: _____

Goals: _____

Warm Up

Activity	Sets	Reps	Time	Dist	Intensity	Note

Core Body

Exercises	Sets	Reps	Weight	Rest Time	Note

Upper Body

Exercises	Sets	Reps	Weight	1RM	Rest Time	Note

Lower Body

Exercises	Sets	Reps	Weight	1RM	Rest Time	Note

Cool Down

Activity	Sets	Reps	Time	Dist.	Intensity	Note